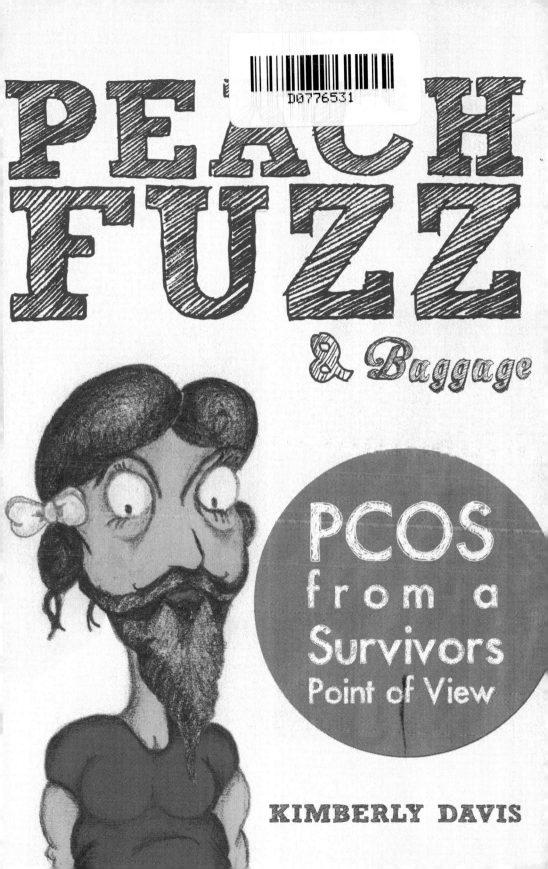

Peach Fuzz and Baggage

PCOS From A Survivors Point Of View

1/1/2013

Kimberly Davis, LVN
AND
P.C.O.S. Survivor

Contents

Forward

Polycystic Ovarian Syndrome is a disorder that has been being diagnosed for about the last seventy-five years, but it seems people and doctors are taking a more active stance in educating themselves about it. With the growing field of reproductive endocrinology and increased education on the subject, more and more women are getting treatment sooner. This is a positive note, when so many women have suffered for so long.

According to the APA Publication: The Lancet, it is estimated that 1 in 15 women suffer from PCOS. The numbers have doubled at an alarming rate and could be possibly linked to the rise in obesity. The effect of this are an increased burden on the healthcare industry; as Type 2 Diabetes, Heart Disease, and other health risks are complications of this disorder.

PCOS is still shrouded in mystery. The links that have been found don't always add up. Medical researchers continue to investigate the causes of the disorder. Women who suffer from it continue to wonder what caused it, if they will ever get pregnant, and if they will ever be cured of PCOS. It often goes undiagnosed for years and, when it is diagnosed, doctors are often quick to put females on birth control hormones to attempt to regulate menstrual cycles. This treatment does not always work and women are still left with questions and the need for support and understanding.

Until an exact cause and cure is found, it is extremely to educate the public on what we DO know about PCOS. It is also extremely important to educate on sound health practices to help control it. Eating a healthy diet, getting plenty of exercise, and early diagnosis and treatment are all important to the best possible outcomes with PCOS. It is also important to understand the factors connected with disorders related to the endocrine system such as viral syndromes, chemical exposure, processed foods, and stress.

The public also needs to understand that PCOS sufferers need a supportive environment to help manage the disorder effectively. There are many physical and emotional complications of PCOS. Many women suffer alone and in silence. Partners and families also suffer right alongside someone with PCOS. PCOS sufferers need to learn how to build a network and a system to help manage this condition both emotionally and physically.

In this three part series, you will be taken through all of the aspects of Polycystic Ovarian Syndrome. This book and its companions will guide you through the causes, symptoms, and all the forms of treatment available, as well as personal insights from a PCOS sufferer and survivor. In a world that lacks understanding and compassion, it is comforting to know that there are others out there who understand what you are going through. In a world of technology, where the internet lacks personal connections in real time, this book is intended to help close that gap.

Let's take a quick look at the books:

Book One "Peach Fuzz and Baggage: PCOS from a Survivors Point Of View" takes you through what PCOS is; the causes, symptoms, emotional impacts, impacts on your life and your body, and treatment options from a medical and natural alternative standpoint.

It is also an in-depth, behind the scenes look at my living with PCOS. It is completely understandable that everyone is different, but you might find some comfort in knowing that someone understands your battle.

There are also "positive quotes" to help lift you up each day. The book also contains illustrations to help you better understand the medical terminology and how the entire endocrine system works.

Included is an appendix with helping links for financial assistance, support groups, and further education on PCOS.

Book Two "Natural Approaches To PCOS: Diet, Alternative Medicine, and Natural Fertility" This book will introduce you to all that you can do to help PCOS naturally. It explains the diet based on The Glycemic Index, Yoga; Meditation, Acupuncture, and natural methods to monitor and improve fertility. It also goes into chemical exposures and the disruption of the endocrine system. There are easy ways to "go natural" without spending a bundle of money. This is everything you need to start taking care of yourself and improving your health with PCOS right at home without medications and is a good route to try if you are on a budget.

Book Three "Modern Medicine and PCOS " This book explains modern medical advances in the treatment of PCOS. It describes fertility drugs, surgical approaches, and the use of anti-diabetic medications to reduce androgens in women. It also helps you to make clear decisions on a plan of treatment and how to create your own treatment plan with both medical and natural approaches to achieve your highest level of health and healthy living. This book also goes into risks and complications and the financial burden.

With education and understanding, PCOS is a highly manageable condition. Having a three part series makes the huge world of PCOS much easier to digest and absorb. Take each book, mark it, print out charts, and use the uplifting mantras to help you on your journey.

Introduction

"Walking with a friend in the dark is better than walking alone in the light." Helen Keller

I am right here holding your hand. There are so many women who have Polycystic Ovarian Syndrome that feel completely alone and lost. That was me. None of my friends, family, or my husband understood what was going on with me. It was a long and very lonely road. I knew I wasn't well, but I looked completely fine on the outside. I actually developed a jealousy for people who felt good. They lived their lives like there was no tomorrow, for me, tomorrow had already come and gone and I was counting the days until I felt better. Feeling better was what I had to look forward to. That positive attitude was only a small glimmer of hope in my darkest hours. I doctor hopped hoping to find an answer. They tested me for every strange and odd disease known to man. The answers to all their testing: Negative. I was labeled a "hypochondriac." I was diagnosed with mental illness. I was even admitted to a mental unit for six days and heavily medicated, for no apparent reason. Except for the fact that I felt so bad, I didn't have the strength to fight anymore. I felt so hopeless and alone. I just needed a doctor who understood my symptoms and what they meant. I had to keep looking and searching for "Doctor Right." No matter how bad I felt, I continued to search.

Now for a little bit about my journey with PCOS. My story is a bit more complicated than most. You see, PCOS is only a part of what I have.

Recently, an endocrinologist put together all of my health issues (mainly endocrine) and diagnosed me with Polyglandular Autoimmune Disease. They are quickly finding that many sufferers of PCOS actually have this and the symptoms are very similar. So, PCOS was more of a co-existing piece of my larger condition.

I suffered from chronic stomach aches as a child. I also suffered from borderline high blood sugar and was tested for diabetes repeatedly when I was little. They just put me on a "low-carb" diet and never looked into it. The stomach aches were diagnosed as gastritis and nothing was ever looked into. Back in the 70s, they really didn't look into much with kids. So, I suffered most of the time as a child. I started my period at a very normal age, thirteen and didn't really have much trouble. I also became a "teen mom" at the young age of seventeen and didn't have any problems getting pregnant. What I did have was those horrid stomach aches during my pregnancy. I also had problems with high blood sugar. But my gorgeous son was born healthy and I went on to finish high school and start my first job.

It all came crashing down at age twenty-three. I was doing well in life with work and my son. I had my own apartment and was very happy. The beginning of my journey happened one morning when I woke up with the worst stomach ache I had ever felt. I was rushed to the emergency room where they diagnosed me with Acute Pancreatitis. I nearly died. I was in the hospital for six weeks on Total Parenteral Intravenous feedings. During this time, they found cysts on my pancreas. My mom also found a rash all over my body that was diagnosed as Tinea Versicolor or Yeast Rash. So, they removed my gallbladder to relieve the strain on the pancreas and I recovered eventually.

At this point, we thought nothing of the previous episode and I felt better. Shortly after my recovery, I relocated to a quiet town in Central California to restart my life, settle down, get married, and start a family. It was a cute little farming town and the people were really nice. I got another apartment and a really good job. Within the first year, I met the man I would one day marry and have kids with. My life was finally going in a good direction!

About a year after we married, my husband and I began to talk about having a baby. We tried just like everyone else, and nothing. As a matter of fact, I never used birth control from the beginning and never once did it cross my mind that I had gone a whole year without getting pregnant. After I thought about it, I knew something wasn't right. My oldest son was conceived so easily.

Although I didn't know yet that I truly had PCOS, I picked up a copy of a book that went over fertility diets and basal temperature charting. I began eating very healthy, charting my temperatures, and just paying more attention to my body. For so long, I ate nothing but fast food and junk food, it was about time for some lifestyle improvements. I learned to eat whole grains, healthy fruits, and vegetables. I took my temperature every morning and recorded any symptoms of ovulation on a chart. I did this for months. It was eleven months to be exact. On Thanksgiving weekend, we had taken a trip to my mother's four hours away in Los Angeles. I felt funny. I was nauseous and I realized that my period might be late. I waited till we got home from our trip and went to see my doctor. That afternoon I got the phone call, I was pregnant. We were so excited!

My pregnancy was everything less than normal, though. It was a hormonal mess if you ask me. I gained far too much weight; I developed pre-eclampsia and high blood sugar levels. My blood pressure was so high they had to give me steroid injections and deliver my daughter almost eight weeks early. She couldn't breathe on her own and had to be placed on a ventilator and taken to a nearby children's hospital for her first week of life. It was like my body was telling me that my body was too unhealthy for reproduction and not to mess with nature. One thing I noted was that at my six-week check-up they found a nodule on my thyroid. They biopsied it and found I had Hashimoto's thyroiditis. An auto-immune condition that often shows up after childbirth and the doctor just wanted to watch it. So we did.

The good news was my daughter ended up being a very healthy baby. She is fifteen years old now and she is amazingly beautiful and smart and she can sing like an angel. It made my struggles in life worth every minute to watch her grow up. I also had a third and fourth blessing come into my life. Shortly after Ashlee was born, I became pregnant with my son Keith. Judging by my diagnosis of PCOS, the remaining pregnancy hormones helped to regulate my body for a while and I conceived naturally without any trouble. My youngest son was born and actually my pregnancy with him was extremely healthy. I thought I was in the clear from health issues and went to nursing school and obtained my degree. The day I got my nursing license was one of the best days of my life.

I started working at a local sub-acute facility taking care of very sick patients on ventilators. It was hard work. I worked the night shift and it felt like I slept all the time. One day, I got sent out of town on a transfer to San Diego. The ride down in the back of the ambulance was uneventful for me. We dropped off our patient, had lunch and then embarked on our six hour drive back home. It was then I noticed something was "off." I started to feel dizzy and unwell. I got back to work and clocked out and went home. I called in sick the next day. I was so dizzy, I could hardly walk. I crawled to the bathroom. When I had a bowel movement, it smelled something like "burnt rubber." I began to have severe heart palpitations, night sweats, severe fatigue, and weight loss. I had to borrow a pair of pants from my oldest son's girlfriend because mine had become far too big. I went from a size 15 to a size 3 in a matter of months.

The doctors tested me for every disease known to man. Every single test was negative. All they could tell me was they thought it was something endocrine. I had horrid pains in my lower right side, but no appendicitis. An ultrasound showed cystic ovaries, but nothing too bad. I was growing hair on my chest and my face. I had chest pain, high blood sugars, and very high blood pressure. Yet, all the lab tests were inconclusive.

I found a really good doctor during my doctor hopping episodes and he felt it did have something to do with my endocrine system. He found me a great reproductive endocrinologist who had me come in for her full battery of lab testing. She called me back in a week later and was 99.9 percent positive that I had Polycystic Ovarian Syndrome. She promptly put me on a popular diabetic drug, Metformin, that helps to control the blood sugars and reduce the incidence of ovarian cysts. I felt better than ever and I began to pick the pieces of myself up and move on with my life.

It had been a rough year and a half from that first dizzy spell until I finally got my diagnosis. I was literally in bed the whole time. I had friends stop by to visit me as if I were some fragile hospital patient. People talked in whispers outside my door. I felt like death was knocking at my door. I could hardly care for my family. But the medication was working and I was finally feeling better. I still could not figure out what it was that made me feel so sick. Only later would I come to find that one of my ovaries had literally rotted and decomposed inside of my body. A condition called "premature ovarian failure," where the ovaries can literally die and atrophy. That was the reason for the horrid smell. I was toxic. The metformin calmed my cysts down and I became pregnant with my fourth and last child, a beautiful daughter. That pregnancy was riddled with problems as with my first daughter. I had to go on insulin injections for gestational diabetes and my blood pressure climbed really high. She was born healthy, but my health continued to deteriorate. They decided within the first year after her birth to do a hysterectomy. It was then that they found the dead ovary. It had indeed atrophied and turned to stone. They found several cysts on it along with several tubal pregnancies in the fallopian tube that had decomposed inside of me, as well. They took my uterus and my cervix with the right ovary and tube. They could not remove the left because it was so cystic and it had developed a large vascular blood supply and the risk of bleeding was high. It served me well, though. It provided me with an extra five year dose of female hormones.

The main disorder I have is Polyglandular Autoimmune Syndrome. They found cysts on my pancreas, my ovaries, and my thyroid. To date, I have donated my gallbladder, my right ovary, and my thyroid to science. My thyroid was removed June 2010 due to cysts. I am on several endocrine replacement medications. I have my good days and my bad days. But, I made it through and now I am here to support and encourage anyone facing PCOS.

From here on out, we will address Polycystic Ovarian Syndrome by its mnemonic, PCOS. And I will start by telling you that the best way to attack PCOS is with education. How did I manage this? I put every symptom in the Google© search bar all at once and PCOS kept popping up. I know it sounds silly. The internet can have very good information or very erroneous information depending on how you look at it. But the odds were I finally had a lead on my diagnosis. What I didn't know, was that my diagnosis was much larger than even that. But, we will get to that in a minute. Let's talk about you.

My hope for you is that this book and the next few in my series give you a solid foundation to begin your journey with PCOS. It is my one dream that PCOS sufferers or someone who knows someone with PCOS will read this book and have that "Ah-Ha" sort of moment. I hope it is that single moment in time where something just falls into place and you feel the comfort of someone who completely understands how you feel. Once I found that moment for myself, I found the strength to stand up and fight. I want to be your friend who walks with your through the darkness, until you feel strong enough to stand on your own two feet. We can giggle together about the effects of the hormonal changes, hence the name of this book. Yes, we have peach fuzz on our faces and a little extra baggage both emotional and physical and I understand where you are.

Disclaimer: This book is not intended for self diagnosis or treatment of PCOS. This condition must be evaluated and diagnosed and the self treatments described should only be done while under the care of a qualified physician.

My name is Kimberly Davis. I just recently relocated from California to New England. My health is too bad to work as a nurse anymore. I am now living out my dream of living in New England as a writer. I have more good days than bad days. I used to be a victim of PCOS and now I call myself a survivor. I have four amazingly beautiful children, a grandchild, and another grandchild on the way. My life is blessed. I hope that through my eyes you can find hope in your own life. Hope to find the right doctor. Hope to find the right treatment. Hope to find the best quality of life in the face of this disease, Polycystic Ovarian Syndrome.

Chapter One

Understanding PCOS From A Survivors Point Of View

"The most beautiful people we have known are those who have known defeat, known suffering, known struggle, known loss, and have found their way out of the depths. These persons have an appreciation, a sensitivity, and an understanding of life that fills them with compassion, gentleness, and a deep loving concern. Beautiful people do not just happen." — Elisabeth Kübler-Ross

When you suffer from Polycystic Ovarian Syndrome, you feel like you live in your own little bubble. For one, you constantly wonder what all of these symptoms mean. You feel as if not one person understands what you are going through. You try and try to explain to your partner, your family, and your friends what this disorder is all about. No one understands. Not even your doctor understands. You are labeled a hypochondriac; you may get misdiagnosed and find yourself doctor hopping only to find dead-ends everywhere you look.

Sound familiar? You're not alone. Millions of women suffer from Polycystic Ovarian Syndrome or PCOS. It is sneaky, often being called a "silent killer." It is brutal on the body and heartbreaking to your emotional state. I know this because I have lived with PCOS for over twenty years. The one thing that brought everything together for me was education. I set out to find any and all information on PCOS, so that I could better understand what was happening to my body. Once the diagnosis was made, I had the tools I needed to deal with my condition more effectively. I also had the tools to better work with doctors, my partner, and family and friends.

It took a lot of work for me and I learned how to deal with PCOS by living with it. I gathered information along the way, but most of my education on this disorder was I had to experience the pain and let downs firsthand. About ten years into my symptoms, I finally became internet savvy. I would put each of my symptoms into the search engine and each time PCOS popped up to the top of the list. The only thing that didn't make sense was the fact that I was having children. There was a twelve year separation between baby number one and baby number two, but with dietary changes and practice I got pregnant three times all by myself, without medical intervention. Baby number four was the product of metformin, but we will talk about that later on in the book. She was a HUGE surprise!

In order to live with PCOS, you first have to understand what is going on with your body. This first chapter will take you through what PCOS is, the symptoms, getting diagnosed, and treatment options. My hope is to prepare you to find the right doctor who understands, make informed decisions in your treatment plan, and learn tools to live healthy for the rest of your life. PCOS management takes commitment and hard work but it is manageable with the right tools. Okay, so let's get started. Without further adieu, here is PCOS from my nutshell.

WHAT EXACTLY IS POLYCYSTIC OVARIAN SYNDROME?

A big huge headache! For most sufferers of PCOS, all they know is that the disorder really puts a wrench into every area of their lives. From checking blood sugars, dieting, ovulation predictors, scheduled lovemaking, failed pregnancy tests, and just feeling generally unwell. I first-off want to set your mind at ease, there is a very good explanation for how you are feeling.

Understand that PCOS is a metabolic disorder that can affect the entire endocrine system. Some people have the misconception that PCOS is cysts on the ovaries. These cysts are actually the normal follicles that develop on the ovaries prior to ovulation and they are not a bad thing. The problem is with PCOS there are too many follicles that do not mature as they should. But the disorder affects much more than just the ovaries. Women with PCOS tend to have high blood sugar, high lipid levels in the blood, hypertension, and higher rates of infertility. It has severe impacts on total body health and longevity if left untreated.

PCOS was first discovered in the 1930s by Irving F. Stein, Sr. and Michael L. Levanthal. The condition was first named *Stein - Levanthal Syndrome*, and the first of their findings concurred that irregular periods were caused by the lack of ovulation. But they realized there was much more research to be done on the actual cause of this disorder and their discovery sparked a new trend to study the relationship of the ovaries and the endocrine system with total body health, genetics, obesity, and other factors. To this day, the research continues and more and more answers to this condition are being found every day. Treatments are improving and the quality of life for many women is improving by leaps and bounds. In order to live with and survive PCOS you need to understand it fully.

The cause of Polycystic Ovarian Syndrome still remains a mystery. There are many factors and clues that help to bring understanding and direction to treatment plans. Truth is, Aunt Edna may hold a key to why you have that or any other endocrine problems. Genetics are one clue and have been found to play a very large role in PCOS or endocrine disease as a whole. Obesity is also a factor, but researchers are still on the fence whether PCOS causes obesity or obesity increases the risk of PCOS. It is a true, "what came first-the chicken or the egg" type situation. I was very thin my entire life until my mid-twenties when I packed on the pounds, right about the same time I noticed I was having fertility problems. I didn't eat any more than normal, but my metabolism seemed to slow way down for no apparent reason. At the time of my actual diagnosis years later, I had actually dropped several pounds and was underweight. Even so, I still noticed that I had a "different" body shape than other women. Smaller on the top, larger at the waist, but we will get into that a little later.

Polycystic Ovarian Syndrome is related to lower levels of sex hormone binding globulin (SHBG) and elevated androgen levels (male hormones). SHBG is a protein that helps to bind certain steroids and has a positive relationship with insulin and thyroid hormones. Hormones are responsible for regulating all of the body's responses and communications. They tell each organ and cells of the body when to function and when not to function. They are essentially messengers. For example, you eat a carbohydrate and the hormone insulin is released and helps the body turn a carbohydrate into glucose and penetrate the cell walls where it is used for energy.

When this hormone pattern is disrupted due to PCOS, the person is said to have "insulin resistance." This happens when androgen excess does not allow the hormone insulin to enter into the cells and provide energy. This is one of the main causes for weight gain and fatigue in PCOS. The blood sugar is often stored as fat when it cannot be properly used for energy and without energy, you feel downright exhausted. Exhaustion keeps us from getting enough exercise and the whole thing becomes a vicious cycle.

The list of hormonal dysfunctions caused by excess androgens is actually quite extensive. Not only does it cause a direct disruption in the ovarian follicles releasing mature eggs and problems with fertility, but this condition can disrupt many of the hormonal processes in the body, like insulin resistance mentioned above. We will take a more thorough look at the hormone communications between endocrine organs a bit later.

Women with PCOS may have a higher inflammatory response in the body. This has been found because women with excess androgens also have elevated levels of C-Reactive Proteins or CRP (inflammation markers) in the body. It was originally thought the increased inflammation was related to obesity, but CRP is elevated in both obese and non-obese women with PCOS. When these levels are elevated, women can experience symptoms such as joint pain, low-grade fevers, headaches, and even colitis. The inflammation response is also a clue to later effects of PCOS. Increased inflammation can cause inflammation of the blood vessels and lead to increased risk of heart disease.

Because of the high levels of inflammation, sebaceous follicles can become inflamed leading to an onset of acne in women with PCOS. Some women with PCOS have complained of adult acne up until their forties. This problem can affect teenagers the most, since they are already dealing with changing skin and bodies during puberty. I am still breaking out with pimples at forty-four years old, but at my age makes me feel like I still retain some youth.

Excess androgens can also cause disruptions in the function of the thyroid and thyroid hormones. On another note, hypothyroidism could be the cause of anovulation itself and not PCOS. This is why a good thyroid work-up is essential to rule out thyroid disease vs. PCOS. However, in cases of PCOS thyroid disease may co-exist at the same time. This was my problem. Not only did I have excessive cysts on my ovaries, I also developed them on my thyroid gland which later had to be removed.

Women who have excessive testosterone levels may experience increased anger. It may even play a role in post-partum depression and mood swings. Studies also show that increased testosterone levels in newborns may play a role in fussy babies. Mood swings may mirror that of a woman going through menopause and can be very hard to control. This is one symptom of PCOS that people around you will take very personally. Truth is, you truly cannot help it when this happens and you don't mean it either.

Other affects are high cholesterol, increased risk of cancer, hypertension, excessive hair growth or loss, and oxidative stresses on the body. PCOS can affect one of these systems or in more severe cases; all of these areas may be experienced. Or, as in my case, there is a whole different set of effects on the body depending on the root cause of the condition. For me, PCOS was just one of many endocrine issues I had to work through since my condition is auto-immune.

There is also a connection in the Cortisol levels with PCOS. Cortisol is a steroid released from the adrenal glands and helps regulate stress, break down glycogen into glucose, and burn carbohydrates. Women with PCOS are shown to have altered levels of Cortisol in their bloodstream. This leads researchers to believe that PCOS also has a connection to the adrenal glands. However, researchers do not think that the increased Cortisol levels are a direct cause of PCOS.

PCOS is a double edged sword so to speak. Higher glucose levels, higher androgen levels, and excess insulin causes the follicles on the ovary's to stop the release of eggs and the cysts themselves can increase production of androgens when the eggs are not released. The good news is an androgen secreting tumor on the ovary can be removed and possibly stop the condition. In most PCOS sufferers, this is not possible because the hyper secretion of androgens come from other areas in the body. There are so many places that excess androgens can stem from.

The first is a malfunction in the pituitary gland. This is a gland located in the brain and signals the release of hormones. Pituitary malfunction is usually caused by a pituitary tumor. The main symptom in this case of PCOS is headaches. The tumor may or may not show up on MRI and only requires treatment if the person wishes to have children. In which case, depending on the size of the tumor, it can either be surgically removed or medications given to try and shrink the tumor.

Tumors, malfunctions, over-production, under-active; it is all still very confusing, I know. It helps to understand how the endocrine system works in detail, because it is a very finely tuned system. Here is a brief overview of endocrinology:

IF YOU NEVER UNDERSTOOD THE ENDOCRINE SYSTEM AND ALL ITS QUIRKS

I never really did either, until I got PCOS. I knew that hormones were connected to my periods and made me cranky around "that time of the month" but I never really knew the mass production going on inside my body that made everything work.

Your endocrine system is your body's main control system. One hormone communicates with another and sends signals to your cells and organs to do their job. The endocrine system is sort of like the "boss," in day to day operations. Each endocrine organ system in the body has its own special set of hormones they both produce and respond too. Think of it kind of like a freeway, the messages are being sent along their way all day long. When the message arrives at its destination, the cells or organs follow the instructions and send messages back on how they are doing. The system can turn off and on as needed based on the messages it receives. You have enough of something, it shuts off. When you need something, it turns on. **(See Figure 1)** This illustration shows each "zone" of the body has its very own control center that links to the main control centers in the brain. Picture lines running from each to zone one another and to the top of the body. The signals actually travel along the same pathways as the nervous system.

The system is very complex and all of the components need to be in communication with each other. As you can see in Figure 1 below, there is an endocrine organ for each organ system in the body. One controls metabolism, one for heart rate and breathing, one for digestion, one for reproduction, one for sleep, and even one for the body's immune system (thymus). They each have their own job to do and they even help each other out.

They can also throw each other off very easily in the process. If there is too much of something and the endocrine organ forgets to shut it off, then somebody was sleeping on the job or got lost on the freeway. Other systems try to compensate, but doing their own job and the work of another system will cause them to tire more easily and start to sleep on the job. Before you know it, you start to feel terrible in every possible way. This is why PCOS sufferers often find themselves on medications for several different conditions. Diabetic medications because the body isn't responsive to insulin, blood pressure medications because the arteries become more narrow from higher blood sugars and lastly, your adrenal glands "burn-out" and your Cortisol is too low to keep up with day to day stresses.

In understanding how the endocrine organs work together, you can try to keep yourself as healthy as possible to prevent strain on other areas of the system. Keeping your blood sugars stable will keep strain off the pancreas. Keeping your weight down may help to lower androgen levels and prevent unnecessary stress on the body to help keep your adrenal glands strong. The whole process in your adrenal system begins at the top and works its way down and then back up.

You have to start with keeping your life as stress-free at possible and get enough rest. Then you have to eat right and drink plenty of healthy fluids. You should switch to decaffeinated coffee or tea and cut out excess processed foods and refined sugars. Keep your body a well-oiled machine and it will be much easier for you in the long-run.

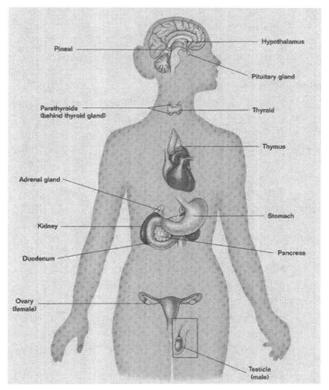

Figure 1: Endocrine System
Photo Courtesy of: epa.gov

It all starts with the "little guy" up top, the hypothalamus; which is the main gland responsible for the signals to the body and the pituitary gland to release hormones. The pituitary gland is also pretty small, but has a very big job. It regulates the sex hormones (androgens in guys and estrogen/progesterone in us girls), thyroid stimulating hormones, growth hormones, and hormones that help to control the kidneys. Hanging out with these guys is the pineal gland; that helps to regulate sleep hormones.

Moving down the body; the thyroid, parathyroid, pancreas, adrenal, ovarian and testicular glands all secrete their own hormones to perform functions in the body. Each has its own job and they all work together like a team.

For instance; your thyroid is an endocrine organ and secretes thyroid hormone to control the body's metabolism. It controls weight, heart rate, blood pressure, temperature, etcetera. When there is not enough thyroid hormone, the body raises a hormone level called your TSH (thyrotopin stimulating hormone). This hormone travels to the thyroid gland and tells it to send out some more thyroid hormone. This is why if you have a "high" TSH level, you're actually "low" on thyroid hormones. If your thyroid is not functioning properly, the body will keep trying to send out more and more TSH to try and get it working again. If your TSH is too high and you don't have enough thyroid hormones for energy, your adrenal glands put out more stress hormones to try and give you extra energy during these "low" periods. Problem is, your adrenal gland can only compensate for this so many times before they start to "burn out." When your TSH is low, then you have enough or too much thyroid hormone. This can also put stress on the body.

This same type of system goes for androgen release, insulin release, steroid release from the adrenal glands, etcetera. The pituitary gland in the brain regulates the control of all of these hormones and gives the endocrine organs instructions on what to do.

One interesting fact is that one androgen; Androstenedione is actually a precursor to estrone, a type of estrogen. This same androgen also converts to testosterone. This steroid is secreted from both the adrenal glands and the testicles in males and ovaries in females. It is right here in this very system that the body seems to allow the production of too much of this hormone and quickly converts it to testosterone instead of estrogen. Studies are still inconclusive as to why, but it seems one of the messengers got off on the wrong exit of the freeway and got lost or just fell asleep on the job.

When that system fails, then you have a problem.

Hormonal imbalances occur for many reasons and PCOS is the result of an imbalance in the steroid hormones in the body including the androgens. Excess androgens block the cells receptiveness to other needed hormones such as insulin. Too many androgens block the sensitivity of the cells to insulin and then the whole endocrine system starts to get out of whack. It is kind of like forgetting to take your car in for a tune-up and then the spark plugs fail and then the engine overheats and then the engine blows up. One problem leads to another. Every system in your body depends on a finely tuned endocrine system.

THE FORGOTTEN "HORMONE" VITAMIN D

I'm now going to throw in a tidbit of my own that may be a little bit controversial, but I may be on to something here. Vitamin D is not something that we take in from food; rather we produce it in our skin when we are exposed to sunlight. Some foods are vitamin D fortified, but it usually isn't enough. After we make or take in vitamin D, our kidneys need to turn it into a form of active vitamin D. Once this happens, it is no longer a vitamin but now a hormone that works to regulate many of the body processes.

Well, in theory Spring Fever is only for animals and not humans. You see, our D levels are higher in the late summer and fall months and drop drastically in the late winter, spring, and early summer months. Studies have shown that estrogen, progesterone, and testosterone are also pretty high in the fall, which makes this our "Fall Fever" and a very optimal time for reproduction. Our bodies are naturally programmed to give birth to babies when our vitamin D levels are higher and our bodies are healthier. That would just about peak in mid-summer. During the cold winter months with less sun, our bodies go into "hibernation" mode. We gain weight, we sleep a lot, and don't have much energy. There is little or no vitamin D passed on to babies from breast milk, so the optimal time to have a baby is in the summer when the baby can make its own vitamin D and mom will have the energy for feeding herself and her baby. One study even showed that women with optimal vitamin D levels had a 47 percent pregnancy success rate with IVF and women with low vitamin D levels only had a 20 percent success rate with IVF.

So, what I am leading up to is in the late fall and winter months through early spring, ovulation may be suppressed to prevent pregnancy naturally and all those follicles still remain as cysts. I always felt worse with my condition during these darker months and I was most fertile in the fall. Three out of my four babies were born smack dab in the middle of summer and one in November. I have now been put on a prescription form of active vitamin D due to my thyroid surgery and it truly has helped me feel better.

Like I said, this is pretty much just in theory and I will outline vitamin D issues in my book on natural alternatives. Turns out, as women we really do need to be getting enough vitamin D for good health. As always, speak to your physician before adding extra vitamin D to your regimen as too much can be toxic.

Now let's talk about that body type issue.

PCOS AND BODY TYPE

Women with PCOS tend to have a different body fat ratio than women without PCOS. This clearly made sense to me after looking at myself in the mirror one morning recently. Women with PCOS tend to have higher fat concentrations in the abdominal region and less in the upper body and breast region. I am quite a bit smaller on the top end, with a rounder middle section. That explains a lot, but why do we get PCOS?

Since PCOS patients are found to have higher than normal levels of androgens in the body, women with PCOS tend to have higher levels of testosterone, androstenedione, DHEAS, and dihydrotesterone (DHT). Many people think that androgens are specifically male hormones but, in all actuality, men have a few female hormones and women have a few male hormones for proper body function. It is these hormones that determine where fat is stored in the body. In men, androgens actually cause them to store less fat and build more muscle tissue and in women it is completely the opposite.

People with balanced levels of androgens store fat lower in the hips and up higher in the chest area. People with androgen excess tend to store fat closer to the middle section of the body. **(See Figure 2)** I am a definite apple shape, but with the glycemic index and keeping my blood sugar levels stable I have managed to retain a "thinner" version of this shape. However, I have to buy my waist size a bit larger to avoid the "muffin top" syndrome in which my fifteen year old daughter teases me about constantly.

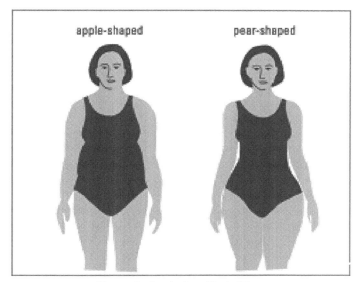

Figure 2: Apple-Pear Body Type
Photo Courtesy of: womenshealth.gov

The PCOS body type is the "apple shape" body and increased belly fat is strongly associated with higher androgen (male hormone) levels. Excess androgens cause higher than normal body fat deposits in certain areas of the body. This body type is also strongly associated with Metabolic Syndrome in men and women, a condition that includes diabetes, hypertension, and high cholesterol.

Having the appearance of the PCOS body type or "apple shape" may strongly suggest that you are at risk for this condition. Do a quick check on yourself to see if your risk is higher according to your waist size. According to the, *National Heart Lung and Blood Institute,* "Waist sizes need to be below >40 inches for men and below >35 inches for women to be considered non-risk for metabolic syndrome." This may also hold true for PCOS sufferers and may be a clue that you need to pay attention to.

Place a measuring tape around your waist above the iliac crest or hip bones. The tape should wrap around about halfway between the lower end of ribcage and top end of the hip bones to be correct. No fair "sucking it in" this time, your measurements won't be correct. Keep your stomach in a relaxed fashion and stand how you naturally would. On the other hand, don't push your stomach out either.

If your measurements are above the guidelines and you are showing symptoms of PCOS, then it is probably time to find a doctor for testing and possibly even treatment. Even if you are not showing any symptoms of PCOS, it is still a good time to make some serious lifestyle and diet changes. Losing a few pounds could lower androgen production, increase your response to insulin, and stop PCOS before it gets started in the first place. Looking back, I wish I had done that before I started having problems. I ate carbohydrates like crazy, didn't drink any water, and never ever exercised. A healthy lifestyle might have been that "ounce of prevention" that I needed.

THE NUMBERS ARE ALARMING

Endocrine disorders as a whole are increasing at an alarming rate. Type I and Type 2 Diabetes are on the rise, as well as Addison's disease (An adrenal gland disorder), Polycystic Ovarian Syndrome, Thyroid Disease, and Parathyroid Disease (Regulates calcium metabolism). Most of these are also caused by autoimmune disorders where the body turns on itself and attacks its own organs and these are on the rise too. It is my humble opinion that this may be the result of exposure to chemicals that "disrupt" the endocrine system functions. Another reason to buy organic whenever possible! This is why in my next book I will thoroughly outline processed foods as endocrine disruptors. I have a whole chapter of information that is really eye opening.

It is estimated that up to ten million American women suffer from PCOS. The numbers could raise a lot higher, since the disorder often goes misdiagnosed or un-diagnosed altogether. That works out to be about 6 to 10 percent of all women. Many PCOS sufferers are misdiagnosed with only Type 2 Diabetes, stand-alone obesity, and Hypertension. Many regular doctors tend to miss the connection. It takes a good reproductive endocrinologist with a carefully trained eye to paint the whole picture.

That is the purpose of this book. I want to reach out to as many women as possible that may be sitting there wondering what is wrong. So many different body systems are affected and each woman is affected differently. I was so confused at what was going on with my body and all the doctor's could tell me was that something was wrong with my endocrine system. From panic attacks to dizziness, high blood sugar, high blood pressure, excess hair growth, and infertility. For me, the clues to my diagnosis came from educating myself. PCOS took thirteen years of my life from me before I received treatment and felt better.

I decided to become your advocate. I firmly believe that with education, more women might see their doctors and be properly diagnosed and receive the proper treatment. More women may be able to have children, lose unwanted pounds, and live healthier lives. The treatment numbers show that after only two-months of proper treatment many women are able to conceive and after six-months of treatment, 90 percent of women with PCOS are back to having normal ovaries, menstrual cycles, and improved endocrine function.

So, the next question is "how do you know if you have PCOS?"

WHAT ARE THE SIGNS AND SYMPTOMS OF PCOS?

Now that I look back, way back in the dark ages; I remember a boyfriend at nineteen years old who used to pluck my "witch hairs" from my chin. I truly believe that is when it all started, but at the time I was too busy learning about life to notice. I also remember other things about that time that seem to fit. I was tired all of the time. I had dizzy spells. I suffered from horrible brain fog. I didn't use contraception and never got pregnant. I was found to have higher than normal blood sugars on several occasions. I went to the doctor, but they never put it all together. "Stop eating so many carbohydrates," they told me. "Get more rest," they would say. "You're depressed," in answer to complaints of brain fog. In my heart, I knew they might be missing something. I was right! It took years of journaling and compiling my symptoms to help that one reproductive endocrinologist come to a conclusion. But, it took work and research on my part to help them understand what was going on with my body. If lab tests are not conclusive, then you will need to meet a certain "criteria list" for diagnosis to be made. That criteria list is made of up symptoms you are experiencing now or have experienced in the past.

The signs and symptoms of PCOS are different for everyone. While one person experiences most of them, another may only have one or two symptoms. Some women may gain weight, while some women, such as me, actually lose weight. Some women may be very ill, while some may not even suspect they have it. It is sneaky. It makes you wonder if you are a hypochondriac or just plain crazy. Nothing seems to fit together and there are a lot of doctors that only see black and white in medicine. PCOS is not black and white.

Here is a pretty comprehensive list of the signs and symptoms of Polycystic Ovarian Syndrome:

▶ **Facial or Chest Hair**

▶ **Acne**

▶ **Irregular Periods**

▸ Infertility (Even after a first or second successful pregnancy; this is known as "Secondary Infertility")

▸ Small Breast Size

▸ "Apple" body shape

▸ Darkened Skin in Armpits, Breasts, Groin, and Neck

▸ Thin Hair

▸ Voice Changes

▸ Ovarian Cysts

▸ Ovarian Pain (Lower Left or Lower Right)

▸ Enlarged Clitoris and Pubic Bone

▸ High Lipid Levels

▸ High Blood Sugar Levels

▸ Hypertension

▸ Weight Gain

▸ Skin Tags

▸ Hashimoto's Thyroiditis (Thyroid Nodules)

▸ Pre-eclampsia (Pregnancy Hypertension)

▸ Miscarriage

▸ Mood Swings (Mostly aggression/anger)

From a personal standpoint, I suffered from several more undocumented symptoms that pointed out an endocrine dysfunction in my body. These have now been proven by a new endocrinologist to be part of a much larger disorder, Polyglandular Auto-immune Syndrome, which is closely related to PCOS. I will save that disorder for a later book, but I will list my other symptoms here for your benefit. This is where some of you might experience an, "ah-ha" moment.

▸ Brain Fog

▸ Dizziness

▸ Memory Loss

▸ Chronic Candidiasis (Yeast Rash) of the skin (Tinea Versicolor)

- Vitiligo (White patches of lost pigment on the skin)
- Chronic Conjunctivitis
- Chronic Pancreatitis
- Endometriosis
- Hashimoto's Thyroiditis
- Gestational Diabetes
- Dry Eyes
- Dry Mouth
- Itchy Skin
- Joint Pain
- Chronic Fatigue
- Severe Anxiety
- Problems regulating Potassium and Calcium levels
- Heart Palpitations
- Depression

In no way am I advocating that these symptoms are truly a part of PCOS, but they are symptoms that confused me and made me constantly wonder what was wrong with me. My actual condition is an autoimmune disorder and many of my above symptoms are related to that condition. The reason I am including the other symptoms is researchers are slowly beginning to find more people that have Polyglandular Autoimmune Syndrome and Polycystic Ovarian Syndrome as coexisting disorders.

It was the coexistence of these two diseases together that made my journey even harder to diagnose and so much to bear for one person. It has been a long road, but knowing the symptoms and being able to pinpoint what I have has made it easier to live with.

THESE SYMPTOMS SOUND ALL TOO FAMILIAR

"We must embrace pain and burn it as fuel for our journey,"
Kenji Miyazawa

If any of the above situations hit home with you, it is time to sit down and have a good think session. Don't panic. Don't be sad. It's not the end of your world. What you need to do first is get a referral to a good reproductive endocrinologist or a regular endocrinologist that may have an interest in PCOS. Now, before you go calling and making any appointments you need to do one very important thing first. Take out a notebook and list every symptom that you have. Whether it is from the above two lists and add in any other physical ailments or symptoms that you have been feeling. This will help the doctor with a diagnosis based on criteria. There are many disorders you can have that don't always come back positive on lab tests. In this case, the doctor will make a diagnosis based on criteria, as I mentioned above.

The most important thing is to gather up strength and not let this part get you down. The worst part of this journey is the unknown. The energy I used up to worry about it from day to day completely burned me out to where I almost didn't have any energy left to fight it once I began treatment. Turn any worries, suffering and bad times into the strength that you will need for the coming months and days. It will benefit you greatly!

And remember, according to the above statistics you are not alone with PCOS. You will begin to find the others; you will find the support and help that you need to hold yourself up on both feet. The first part is the hardest part and you will notice the closer you get to your path for treatment and recovery, the better you will begin to feel inside and out. Connecting with people who feel the same way you do and experience the same symptoms will help to take away that helpless and lost feeling that you may be suffering from. That is exactly how I felt; helpless and lost.

I think a lot of my own suffering was emotional, rather than physical. There was a ton of frustration with trying to get pregnant. All while feeling physically ill and the emotional repercussions to not feeling good enough to have a life really brought me down. Every time a new symptom pops up, you feel let down. It seemed like that happened to me every time I started to feel good again, I would take another step backward and feel down again. You literally spiral up and down, down and up again. It is a physical and emotional roller coaster ride that you wished you didn't have ticket for. Roll with the punches here, girls. Because I didn't have the support system of other sufferers, I didn't read any books written in personal format and my doctors didn't understand; it took me four-long years to know why I felt the way I did. Now, when the symptoms pop up I can tolerate them better. I still don't have much of a support group, but I have the understanding I need to get through. You will too!

COMPLICATIONS OF PCOS

Left untreated, PCOS can wreak havoc on your body. I know this first hand. I didn't know what I had for nine years and only received treatment for two years prior to my hysterectomy. After my hysterectomy, my surgeon came in to tell me he had never seen an ovary so atrophied before in all his years of experience. It had literally turned to "stone." There were several follicles that had broken free and I had several tubal pregnancies that never made it and atrophied in my right fallopian tube (This was due to endometriosis). My left ovary had developed its own vascular system and he had to leave the ovary because of the risk of bleeding. I now have to go through menopause twice, which I am well into my second bout of menopause right now. I had surgical menopause after the hysterectomy and now, five years later, the ovary that was left is now dying out. I am also experiencing hypertension again and some spikes and dips in my blood sugars. I am lucky; it could be worse but isn't too bad this time around. Well, except for those darned nasty "hot flashes." Nothing like waking up drenched and throwing the covers off only to find you also have "cold chills" at the same time you are feeling like you are burning up. I once steamed up only the car windows on my side of the car, all while trying to strip off my coat from under my seatbelt in the middle of winter. My teenage daughter and her friends were laughing so hard at my antics!

The dangerous complications of untreated PCOS are far worse than simple hot flashes during menopause and can include full-blown Type 2 Diabetes, heart disease from increased lipid levels in the blood, damage to the organs, nerves and blood vessels from untreated high blood sugar, ovarian atrophy, and stroke from untreated hypertension and permanent infertility. Some of these complications can happen very early in middle age, with some women beginning cardiac disease in their forties. This should be a time you enjoy, instead of starting multiple medications. They say, "70 is the new 30," meaning that the average human is staying younger longer and enjoy a longer life. PCOS sufferers can too with proper treatment and health maintenance practices. But you have to start working on this early and you have to stick with it. Feeling better, getting pregnant or regular periods are not necessarily the end of PCOS. You will need to continue what works for you even if you get better.

Many of these complications can be avoided with just a change in diet early on in the disease. But, certain measures need to be taken to reduce the amount of androgens in the body and most of the time this does require some form of treatment and cannot be ignored. If caught early enough, the body can be brought back into balance. For some, treatment many need to be continued long-term. As I said above, stick with the diet and exercise plan for the rest of your life to help prevent complications. Keeping androgen levels lower in women protects the arteries and improves insulin response. There is one important reason that androgens need to be kept under control: inflammation.

As discussed earlier, androgens increase inflammation in the body. Inflammation is one of the main causes of circulatory disease. It causes the arteries to harden and form plaque. High cholesterol builds up and makes them even smaller. This in turn leads to high blood pressure and decreased blood flow. Increased inflammation is a recipe for disaster if left untreated or unmanaged. I was lucky that my blood tests for inflammation have all been normal so far. It is a good idea for you to have them checked at least periodically if your initial tests are negative. I have my Sedimentation Rate and C-Reactive Proteins checked at least yearly during my annual physical. Prior to my hysterectomy, my Sedimentation rate was elevated and showed I had some mild inflammation, but after my hysterectomy the levels have been completely normal.

As for complications, I am one of the lucky ones. I was blessed with four children and the after effects aren't too bad, yet. Experts say the risk of complications from PCOS is higher after menopause. I'm still somewhere stuck in the middle of menopause and it can drag on for as long as it needs too. My blood tests still show that I have plenty of estrogen and progesterone in my body and I need those to protect my health. Yes, I still get really painful cysts on my left ovary but I know that the fact it functions is good for me. So, it is important to keep up your regular visits with a gynecologist, internal medicine physician, and possibly continue with a reproductive endocrinologist for check-ups.

I see my endocrinologist every six-weeks and my gynecologist every few months to monitor my cysts and get a full work-up done by my internal medicine doctor yearly. So far so good. My cholesterol is lower than normal; blood sugar and blood pressure are all in good ranges. The only issue I continue to have is the cysts on my remaining ovary. This requires periodic ultrasounds to make sure they are not getting larger. They are painful, but no complications so far. I also have to deal with the effects of my Polyglandular Autoimmune Syndrome, but if I can keep my PCOS in check that is much less I have to deal with.

PCOS AND AGE RELATED EFFECTS: WHAT TO WATCH FOR

PCOS can strike anytime at any age. It is a glitch in the endocrine/metabolic processes of the body and why it happens we still don't know. If I had known then what I know now maybe I could have obtained proper treatment early on and not suffered so badly. Hindsight is 20/20, as they say. I am still unsure when my PCOS developed. I may have shown signs in childhood, but back in the early seventies they didn't check kids for much for complicated endocrine conditions. Not unless it was something black and white and straight out of a textbook. My mom would take me to the doctor as a small child and they would monitor my blood sugars. I was a borderline diabetic as a child, but nothing more than normal. I was a very small build and didn't really gain much weight. But there was nothing to actually diagnose me with any kind of endocrine disorder. I only suffered from slightly higher than normal blood sugars. Maybe I had some sort of precursor as a child, maybe not. All I remember is a rash on my body (Candidiasis) and a lot of stomach aches.

Now that I have done my homework and learned a few things, I wanted to compile information on the effects of PCOS during all of the stages of life. This will help both mothers of teenage daughters and daughters of older mothers to have the information needed to address the issue of PCOS. It will also give you the sufferer the information you need at whatever stage of life you are at. You may be twenty and think you have PCOS or you could be fifty and wondering if this is what is wrong with you. Or, you may be somewhere in between and unable to conceive or generally just don't feel right.

PCOS in Childhood According to *The Journal Of Clinical and Endocrinology & Metabolism,* risk factors for Polycystic Ovarian Syndrome can be identified in childhood. The signs tend to be subtle, but do exist and can help with early diagnosis and treatment to prevent complications later in life.

Children at risk for PCOS show signs of endocrine dysfunction such as low birth weight, premature growth of pubic or facial hair prior to eight years old, early sexual development (precocious puberty), obesity, and adrenal disorders. They can also have insulin resistance early on that may require treatment with an anti-diabetic agent. Pediatric endocrinologists can work children up for androgen excess and decide on a course of treatment.

This didn't happen in earlier years and I often wonder if I had been treated for those marginal blood sugars in childhood, maybe my ovaries would have developed properly. Children today have an advantage with new advances in medicine and may be able to avoid issues with proper treatment.

This is why proper diet and exercise is so important for children. Diets that are abundant in fats and simple sugars can cause a whole range of problems in children including high blood pressure, Type 2 Diabetes, and increased cholesterol levels. Childhood obesity is on the rise and overall we need to do something to improve children's health as a whole.

I remember growing up on Campbell's© soups, Chef-Boyardee©, and McDonald's© Happy Meals as a kid. My grandmother babysat me and she had the endless kitchen full of "kid-friendly" foods. I drank gallons of Kool-Aid© and ate cookies and chips for snacks. It wasn't my grandmother's fault, by all means. Kids just ate whatever they wanted back then and no one thought about it. Even school lunches were unhealthy. Today, we have finally taken the initiative to change the diets of children and improve health from the start of life.

PCOS in Adolescence The one main sign of PCOS in adolescence is the lack of ovulation or irregular periods. Teenagers with PCOS also have excessive acne, patches of darkened skin, and weight gain. This can lead to added emotional effects that puberty already deals out. No young girl wants to have to deal with acne or facial hair growth. Weight gain could also pose a serious emotional issue for teenage girls. Finding a pediatric endocrinologist at the first signs of PCOS in teens can help control the symptoms and help keep the condition bearable. It may even prevent ovarian atrophy and infertility later in the childbearing years.

The most important step for young girls with signs of PCOS is to get plenty of exercise and proper diet. If anyone between the ages of twelve and eighteen have two or more signs and symptoms of PCOS, it is important to consult with a physician for a detailed evaluation. Teenage girls with PCOS will need to have their blood sugar tested every year, a glucose tolerance test every two years, and refrain from smoking if using birth control pills to regulate periods. This is the age when PCOS education needs to begin. It is also important for mothers and daughters to have open lines of communication. Many girls feel too embarrassed to tell their caregivers they are having reproductive health problems.

One easy way to remedy this problem is to have teenage girls keep a calendar or datebook and mark the beginning and end of their monthly period. They can also journal other symptoms such as; increased acne, facial hair growth, and weight gain. They can be allowed to keep the book private and only show it to their doctor during check-ups. I do this with my fifteen year old daughter and it gives her a great sense of independence in life. Plus, we can track her symptoms to make sure she is not showing signs of PCOS, which she is not at this time. Whew! I am also very lucky that my daughter craves healthy foods, doesn't really like much junk foods, and she loves to exercise.

PCOS in Child Bearing Years (20's to 40's) Give or take a few years, these are the most important time for good health. PCOS during these years is again a "double edged sword." Dealing with health issues such as; high blood sugar, high cholesterol, and weight issues can be enough. Add in the problem of irregular periods and no ovulation and you may have a tough time. It's never too late to start treatment for PCOS and the sooner the better during these years.

The emotional trauma of PCOS during childbearing years is probably the highest. Women who want to have children, but cannot due to the diagnosis, will have to brace themselves for the "rollercoaster ride" of their lives. Some may have an easy time conceiving and for some conception may be very difficult. This is an important time to have a support system in place. Whether it is fellow PCOS sufferers, survivors like me or trusted friends and family, support is what is going to get you through this period of your life.

For women who do not choose to have children, this time can be just as tough emotionally. Hormones are at their peak during this time in your life, so PCOS is too. You may face emotional challenges from the symptoms and the health issues that arise. I remember when this was bad and I had the most wonderful neighbor that understood and was there for me. There were others that helped hold me up during those years and without them, it would have been so much harder. From one new symptom to another, each day was an emotional challenge and let down. It was good to have people who cared during these tough times for me.

I also cannot stress enough the importance of journaling during the childbearing years. Writing down cycles, symptoms, basal temperatures, medications taken, and medical appointments will make a huge difference in how you deal with PCOS right now. Life gets busy and you have to make time for yourself and your daily journal. It will pay off months down the road when you need to remember the different things you experienced and need to tell your doctor. It will also show response to treatment and you will be able to see how far you have come!

During this time I cannot stress enough the importance of lifestyle changes. Even though you are dealing with PCOS in childbearing years, you still may be planning a pregnancy. Now is the time to quit smoking, cut down on caffeine or switch to decaffeinated coffee, and drink alcohol only in extreme moderation. It will be during the first twelve weeks of a pregnancy that any of these things can affect your growing baby. Many times you will notice in the news about "baby bump" rumors with celebrities because they were seen drinking water and shunning alcohol or caffeine only later to find out they weren't actually pregnant, yet. This is proof that many people change lifestyle habits prior to becoming pregnant. The reason I stress this is women with PCOS have a higher rate of miscarriage and this can happen before you even know you are pregnant.

The Menopausal Years This is the time in a woman's life when years of untreated or undertreated PCOS can have profound effects on total body health during and after menopause. If you have not already been evaluated and treated for PCOS and have symptoms, it's still not too late. While doctors may argue that PCOS ends after menopause is complete, the effects on the cardiovascular system may still be evident and cause a significant higher risk of death in women. It is true that the ovaries may shut down and the androgen levels drop, but hardening of the arteries due to excessive androgens and high blood sugars continues to be present. This is why early treatment is important to reduce the risks of complications later in life.

There are still emotional effects in the menopausal years of PCOS. Coupled with the effects and emotions that come with aging in general, you get a whole other set of emotions to deal with. I am at this phase of life now and it has been hard. For one, I am divorced and reconnected with a childhood sweetheart I have known thirty years. I had a hysterectomy and even though I was blessed with four beautiful babies, there is always the heartache that we cannot have one together. Then, of course, there is still the fact that I have to deal with one ovary that decides when and where to give me a blast of hormones. This has led to some severe menopausal mood swings. Some days, I just want to hide my head under a pillow and not come out. I get through it and I have my good days and my bad days.

The life stages of PCOS are very real. Watching children for early signs of endocrine disease could mean easier childbearing years. Childbearing women who receive treatment early will most likely conceive and be healthier later in life with a lower risk of complications to general health. In the menopausal years, women can take extra good care of themselves to prevent the long-term complications mentioned.

I wish now that my pediatrician had noticed that my borderline high blood sugars and skin discolorations in childhood might have been an indication of what was to come. They didn't go deeply into endocrine disorders in children back then. Things were black and white, you either had diabetes or you didn't. At least now in my peri-menopausal years I really need to take the needed steps to prevent further damage to my body with healthy diet and exercise.

The good thing is I can help my girls to try and stay healthy. I had a rough time with my childbearing years, but I can now take better care of myself during my menopausal years and hopefully stay healthier because of what I have learned.

Chapter Two

The Physical Affects of PCOS

THE DEVASTATING PHYSICAL IMPACT OF PCOS

"I don't think of all the misery, but of the beauty that still remains." Anne Frank

My partner still leans over to me every once in a while and plucks a stray hair from my chin. He thinks nothing of it. He still tells me I'm beautiful. I don't feel beautiful when he does that. It has been a struggle with PCOS to feel beautiful with some of these symptoms. But understanding my condition has made it so much easier to deal with. Lucky for me, he thinks I am beautiful no matter what. Whether it is inner beauty or just what radiates from within, I find something good to celebrate about myself every day.

Some of the physical impacts of PCOS aren't totally devastating, but they can be downright embarrassing. Like, having your partner who thinks you are the most beautiful woman on earth reach over to pluck a hair from your chin. Now that's love! Other symptoms are a little bit of work such as checking your blood sugars regularly and skipping dessert when you adore cheesecake or ice cream. In addition, regular blood pressure checks are also important. Things like that you can work with and live with. It is the devastating physical effects such as obesity, infertility, increased risk of hysterectomy, and the effects later in life that are the biggest hurdles to deal with.

I know this firsthand because I dealt with the disappointment of trying to have a baby. I dealt with the negative pregnancy tests, late periods for no reason, the weight gain, and diabetes with hypertension that almost kept me from working at a career that I loved. My relationship suffered because of scheduled lovemaking and I could tell my partner suffered a lot of emotional let downs right with me. My body was not working right and doctors could not find anything to help me feel better. Needing a hysterectomy by age thirty-eight is not the norm by all means. I was blessed with four children but hysterectomies mean the end of childbearing. There is only one word I can think of: Devastating. Even though I am not having any more children, there is still that feeling that you have lost something as a woman after you have a hysterectomy. That was a whole new set of emotions to overcome for me. With the ovary that they left, I still have to deal with the occasional un-ruptured follicles that give me that all-too-familiar pain in my side. A reminder that PCOS is still a part of my life in some way is the fact that last ultrasound they told me my ovary looked like "a bunch of grapes."

Let's take a look at some of the physical effects that are pretty life changing:

IRREGULAR PERIODS AND INFERTILITY

You wake up and realize your period is late. You run right out to the drugstore and grab, not one, not two, but three pregnancy tests. You want to be sure, right? You take the first one, negative. You take the second one, negative. Three times and they are all negative. As a matter of fact, I'm guessing you probably keep at least one pregnancy test under your bathroom sink at all times? I did and people would laugh at me.

Three tests, all negative and you wonder how you could be two weeks late and yet, not pregnant. I learned that with PCOS the timing of my cycles was a little bit longer than the normal twenty-eight days. (**See Figure 3**) My cycles were actually thirty-five to thorty-seven days long. **This is a key point to remember because later on in my series, I will teach you how to calculate ovulation based on YOUR cycles and not the "textbook" cycles you have been taught.** With PCOS, it is really hard to tell when you ovulate and often hard to tell if a period is an actual "missed period" or lack of ovulation the previous month. Lack of ovulation means you didn't actually get pregnant and you may even miss your period or it may be super late. You are officially in limbo. You have to get to know your cycles like a book.

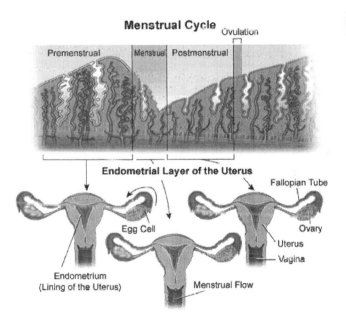

Figure 3: Normal Menstrual Cycle
Photo Courtesy of: yalemedicalgroup.org

PCOS causes irregular periods and it can be really hard to keep track of your cycles. An average menstrual cycle is twenty-eight days and ovulation usually occurs on or about day fourteen. Well, in textbook cases anyways. The most fertile period is a seventy-two hour window occurring the day before ovulation, the day of ovulation, and the day after. In a perfect world this is actually a lot of time for conception because if your partner is healthy, so are his sperm. Healthy sperm live about seventy-two hours under average conditions. In a very healthy vagina and uterus, healthy sperm have been known to survive up to five days. But for a PCOS sufferer that may have acidic levels in the vagina, sperm may only last twelve hours. With ovulation prediction, you almost have to be precisely right on and cannot miss a single step or you have to wait a whole month longer to try.

In PCOS, cycles can stretch out extra days, weeks or even months for some women. This makes it very hard to predict that ovulation window. Ovulation is what makes everything happen to get the body ready for pregnancy. If ovulation does not occur, neither does the buildup of the uterine lining to be ready for pregnancy. If an ovary is polycystic, it may take longer for the mature eggs to break free, or they may not even break free at all. The term I like to use is "sleepy ovaries," because they just don't seem to wake up and respond to the body's signals to do what they are supposed to. The only way to know when ovulation occurs is to track cycles in PCOS by using a chart **(See Figure 4)** and basal thermometer every single day. During the menstrual cycle, the body temperature shifts ever so slightly first thing in the morning right before we awaken. In order to catch this shift, we have to take our temperatures before we move any muscles and cause our temperature to rise. When we are on our period, the temperature stays around the normal body temperature. When ovulation is imminent, the basal temperature drops a steep dip and then rises slightly above the normal body temperature at the time of ovulation. The steep dip tells you to be ready and start trying. If conception occurs, the body temperature will remain slightly high from then on out. If conception did not occur, it will return to normal just prior to the next expected period.

I will also teach you how to check cervical mucus for signs of ovulation and the best environment for sperm to live in. Cervical mucus is the transportation vehicle for sperm to move up the vaginal canal, through the cervix and up through the uterus to the fallopian tubes. The vaginal PH has to be alkaline and the mucus needs to be like "egg-white" consistency. Proper cervical mucus is thin, clear and sort of "stretchy" when placed between two fingers and pulled apart. Cervical mucus that does not support healthy sperm travel is milky, thickened, sticky, or even dry. It is important to check cervical mucus daily when you check your basal temperature, with the exception of when you are on your period. Then you will just note bleeding on your chart. The chart below doesn't depict the letters, but you can use B=Blood, S=Sticky, or T/S=Thin/Stretchy. You can use your own variations and note them on the bottom of your basal chart. You will then be able to note the classic drop in temperature and the Thin/Stretchy mucus on the same day and know you are, in fact, ovulating. It is the hormone estrogen that causes cervical mucus to thin and become ready for sperm travel. PCOS can quickly change estrogen into testosterone and the mucus does not follow the basal temperatures. This makes tracking ovulation hard, but keeps at it, in order to catch this narrow margin; you must accurately take your temperatures and chart your cervical mucus. It's funny, I go back and look at those ovulation charts every once in a while to relive those good feelings of when they actually worked and I became pregnant. They become a nice memento to put in your baby's keepsake box. Yes, I even kept the positive pregnancy test (gross) and those first ultrasound pictures. I guess for me those together were proof that I had overcome something much larger than I imagined and looking back was a source to keep going forward.

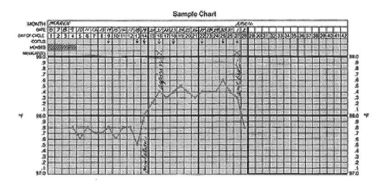

Figure 4: Basal body temperatures and ovulation
Photo Courtesy of: library.med.utah.edu

In **Figure 4** above, you can see how your body temperature from the day you start your period (Day 1) through day 12 is rather steady. On Day 13 you see a dip (pre-ovulation) and then a spike above all of the other temperatures on Day 14 and then the temps stay elevated. On Day 29 the temperatures drop back down showing that the next period is likely about to start.

There is no promise of pregnancy with PCOS. But, with a little effort infertility rates are not as high as people once thought. True infertility is actually quite rare. If you have a uterus, ovaries, and fallopian tubes, your chances of pregnancy are actually pretty good! It just takes more work to get pregnant and sometimes more money than you have. This is the frustrating part, you find yourself wishing that nature would make it happen just as easily as everyone else. Using the basal chart may make that wish come true!

Yes, you can get pregnant with PCOS. But, I need to be brutally honest with you about one thing; there is an increased risk of pregnancy loss with PCOS. If ovaries are a bit slow in releasing the egg, the follicle they were released from may also be a bit slow in releasing needed hormones to sustain the pregnancy in the beginning. When conception occurs, the follicle where the egg was released secretes progesterone. In women with PCOS, the follicle may not secrete enough progesterone or none at all. This can keep the fertilized embryo from implanting in the uterine lining resulting in pregnancy loss. There have been some trials of progesterone replacement therapy in early pregnancy, but studies are showing that there is no evidence of increased success rates with progesterone replacement.

Women with PCOS are also at a higher risk for pregnancy complications including gestational diabetes, pre-eclampsia, and a higher Cesarean section rate because of larger babies. These factors can multiply the devastation of PCOS. I actually made it through three PCOS pregnancies, suffered the complications of pre-eclampsia in one and gestational diabetes in another. It took a little extra work and I have to admit that when my oldest daughter was born, seeing her carted off to the NICU was not a fun experience. I thought I was going to lose her. She was in severe respiratory distress from being delivered early due to my pre-eclampsia. After a week in the NICU on a ventilator she finally came home to us. It was frightening! In my fourth pregnancy, my blood sugars were really high and taking insulin injections twice daily was hard. The extra effort was worth it, but it wasn't easy for me, my partner and my new babies.

I suffered through the complications with three of my pregnancies with PCOS. I wanted children. Because of this, I had a large amount of guilt. Especially for my oldest daughter who was born early and very ill her first week of life. So guilt is another emotion that we sometimes have to deal with. We ask ourselves if it is actually selfish to want children with PCOS. The answer is NO, absolutely not. If you want children and are able to conceive even with help, then you will be able to weather whatever goes along with those pregnancies. Your children will not blame you. They won't even remember. What it was for me was a lesson learned to watch my daughters for the subtle clues that may signal PCOS for them in their late childhood to teen years and then we can get a thorough evaluation early on in the game. I can be a good mother and feed them well and encourage them to exercise. Most of all, I can teach them how to find the strength to get through it if they need it. Hopefully they won't have to.

METABOLIC SYNDROME AND PCOS

This is the part of PCOS that causes effects on the other body systems other than reproductive. The diabetes, hypertension, high lipid/cholesterol levels, and possibly even blot clots are all part of a metabolic syndrome. Metabolic syndrome can happen to anyone with or without PCOS. Not all PCOS sufferers have metabolic syndrome, but there has been a direct link found between PCOS and metabolic syndrome. In cases of metabolic syndrome the one common link that researchers have found is: Insulin Resistance.

This is the part where elevated androgen levels come into play. Elevated androgens block the proper processes of the body's hormonal system and make it go awry. As discussed in the first chapter, androgens keep the hormones from penetrating cell walls and they cannot do their job properly.

Here are some of the effects of Metabolic Syndrome associated with PCOS:

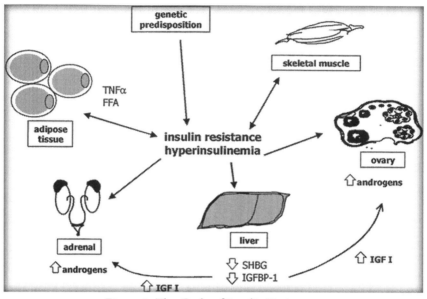

Figure 5: The Cycle of Insulin Resistance
Photo Courtesy of: edrv.endojournals.org

Insulin resistance is still being widely studied. When we eat, our pancreas secretes insulin to help the glucose in our food get into the cells and give us energy. When we have insulin resistance, our body does not use the insulin to allow the glucose into the cells and the glucose stays in the bloodstream and causes high blood sugar levels. It also causes excessive levels of insulin to remain in the bloodstream (Hyperinsulinemia). In turn, hyperinsulinemia affects the liver, the ovaries and the fat cells in the body. It can also stimulate the ovaries to produce even more androgens. **(See Figure 5 Above)** This happens in conjunction with excess androgen levels already present in the body and it is critical that both the androgens and the insulin levels need to be brought back into balance.

Hyperglycemia or high blood sugar is any fasting a.m. blood sugar over 100/ml fasting and higher than 140/ml two hours after a meal. The average population has a fasting blood sugar that is 70 to 80 fasting. In PCOS, the blood sugars are not often high enough to constitute a diagnosis of diabetes and other tests may need to be run by the endocrinologist to show insulin resistance. An insulin level is usually run with blood sugar levels and in PCOS insulin is usually elevated.

Obesity is one factor that researchers are really looking into as a potential cause of PCOS. The theory shows that women who are modestly overweight suffer from excess androgens (male hormones) in their system. Weight reduction seems to bring on a relief of symptoms. The question that does unanswered here: Why do women who are not overweight suffer from symptoms of PCOS?

The answer may lie in the very cysts on your ovaries. What happens is in women with PCOS, the very cysts themselves begin to secrete androgens (male hormones) in higher levels than normal. It has been found that excessive androgen production in any female can lead to insulin resistance. In the same theory, hyperinsulinemia or too high of insulin levels from insulin resistance can also turn around and cause the ovaries to overproduce androgens.

Weight can fluctuate from time to time over the childbearing years. From being moderately overweight to underweight, many women find that their weight tends to be on a rollercoaster ride just like their emotions. This can lead to diet failures and fad dieting in any attempt to control a weight issue. Once the PCOS responds to treatment and the androgens stabilize, many women find the weight tends to melt away. Others may find that it never goes away. It is how you treat yourself with proper diet and exercise that makes all the difference in the world.

Hypertension is another issue with PCOS. Women who suffer from PCOS have higher than normal blood pressures. Studies show that early on in PCOS, the androgen excess has an effect on the renin-angiotensin mechanism in the kidneys. This is the mechanism the kidneys use to balance electrolytes and regulate blood pressure. Women with PCOS may often suffer from imbalances of sodium, potassium, and calcium levels. This is why younger women with PCOS sometimes experience hypertension and need to be treated. Another good reason to chart your blood pressures!

Because of this, there is an importance issue to balance mineral and electrolyte intake. It also means gaining control of excess androgens to help reduce blood pressure and stabilize the kidneys to do their work in regulating fluids properly.

Normal blood pressure is classified as anything under 130/85. Ideally, doctors like to see blood pressures lower than 120/80. If your blood pressure is higher than 140/90, then you are considered hypertensive and may need treatment.

Later on in life, PCOS related hypertension can be due to blood vessel damage from hormones. Arteries can become thickened and narrowed due to high lipid levels, androgens, and high blood sugars. Getting a handle on PCOS before this problem develops can reduce the risk of cardiovascular disease in women later in life.

High Cholesterol is caused by insulin resistance. When there are abnormally elevated levels of insulin floating around in the bloodstream tends to stimulate androgen production by the ovaries and this leads to increased levels of triglycerides and cholesterol. With PCOS, you will need to have your cholesterol checked on a regular basis. PCOS contributes to cardiac complications and it is extremely important to eat a healthy diet and stick to a treatment plan. As stated above, this issue can contribute to smaller than normal arteries and blood vessels and increase the risk of cardiac complications from PCOS.

You will want to try and keep your cholesterol levels in the following ranges:

Total Cholesterol – Below 200 mg/dl

LDL (Low Density Lipoprotein) – Below 70 mg/dl

HDL (High Density Lipoprotein) – Above 60 mg/dl (This is your "good" cholesterol)

Triglycerides - Below 150 mg/dl

I still continue to eat on the glycemic index scale and last time I had my cholesterol checked it measured low cholesterol or "low cardiac risk." Yes, I cheat and eat a bowl of ice cream every now and then. But gone are the days where I eat a half gallon every few days. I limit myself to a bowl of ice cream weekly. I also use fats sparingly and eat plenty of whole grains.

COMPLICATIONS AFTER MENOPAUSE

This is probably the most detrimental effect of PCOS on the body. Years of androgen excess, insulin resistance, high blood sugar levels, high cholesterol, and hypertension can have a profound effect on the body. Yes, these things are a part of getting old, but PCOS sufferers have an increased risk of complications of stroke, heart attack, and kidney disease in later years.

Women who suffer from excessive androgen production can experience some of the same aging effects of androgens that men do. Thinning hair and male-pattern baldness are both complications of PCOS in women. When these symptoms develop, it shows that there is an increased risk from other complications of androgen excess and you may be heading down a dangerous path.

Years of higher than normal blood sugar breaks down the walls of delicate veins and blood vessels. It can even cause damage to the nerves in the feet and legs. If the condition is severe enough, there is a risk of amputation because of damage caused by blood sugar. The kidneys have very delicate blood vessels and prone to damage from high blood sugar. People who suffer from severe diabetes may end up on dialysis due to kidney failure later in life.

When your cholesterol is too high and your blood sugar is too high, paired with the inflammatory response to androgens, your arteries can begin to form plaque buildup and lead to hypertension and increased risk of blood clots, heart attack, and stroke.

Not that aging in general doesn't carry these risks, but with PCOS the risk is much higher because of the damage excess androgens can do to the body. This is why it is best to seek a diagnosis early on when you first experience symptoms, so you can start treatment and live a healthy life.

CONCLUSION

The sum of this chapter is the fact that PCOS can have some small annoying affects on your physical wellbeing, but it can also have some profoundly devastating effects on your health if left untreated. It can also affect your emotional health, your relationships and your career. This is why it is very important to address PCOS as early as possible and begin to treat it before complications develop.

Getting treatment to lower blood sugar, blood pressure, and keep weight to a healthy level should be a first priority with PCOS. Avoiding complications to your physical health is just as important as having a baby. Addressing emotional and relationship issues early on will help keep you strong emotionally and help you avoid the "rollercoaster" ups and downs that PCOS brings with it. Hopefully, you will also be able to recognize the symptoms early on and bring them to your physician's attention.

Most often getting the proper treatment for PCOS will increase your chances of becoming pregnant, having healthy pregnancies, a healthier baby, and a healthy mommy. If you do not choose to have children, you will give your body what it needs to function properly and avoid serious complications in your later years.

Keep journaling your symptoms. Keep charting your cycles. Journal your daily feelings about PCOS and keep the complications that can arise in the back of your mind, but don't allow worries to overcome you. You may feel physically unwell some days and you will have some good days too. Celebrate those good days so you can save up the energy to deal with the bad days. The single most important thing is to keep in touch with your doctors if any new symptoms develop or you notice a significant decline in your physical health.

Chapter Three

PCOS And The Effects On Your Emotional Well-Being

"If you have fear of some pain or suffering, you should examine whether there is anything you can do about it. If you can, there is no need to worry about it; if you cannot do anything, then there is no need to worry." -Dalai Lama

I have spent the greater part of my years worrying about my illness. I have let life pass me by while I focused on finding a doctor that could help me. I canceled dinners with friends, missed the kid's school functions and avoided going outside in the sunshine. All because I didn't feel well and I worried about it constantly. Worrying about my illness did absolutely nothing to make it better. Worrying didn't find me the right doctor. Worrying did not serve me in the least little bit. What I needed to do was find the best quality of life for myself right where I was at with my illness. So, I decided that I wasn't going to stop living for PCOS. I wasn't going to let it control my life anymore. I had to realize that I was in control, not my condition. Somehow, after years of emotional suffering, I learned to live again!

Recently, my boss noticed I wasn't feeling well at work and wondered why I even bothered coming in. I told her that at this point in my illness and my life, I have chosen to live my life regardless of how I am feeling. No longer do I allow myself to be confined to bed. No longer do I cancel on my friends. I don't call in sick to work unless I have a fever. No longer do I worry about my health. It is what it is and I have chosen to have quality of life at whatever level of functioning I am at. Yes, sometimes I feel like staying in bed. Sometimes I want to throw in the towel and let my condition have its way. We all do that sometimes. It is finding the strength to overcome and get moving again that is the key to a good life with PCOS.

I decided to begin the chapters of my book with quotes. I like quotes and I believe in the power of positive thinking. PCOS can have a profoundly devastating effect on not only your physical health but also your emotional well-being. Contrary to popular belief, the emotional toll doesn't always come from not being able to get pregnant. We are women and we want to feel beautiful and good about ourselves. Emotional effects come from several different areas of PCOS.

I have plaques with quotes like these all over my house. They serve me well and remind me every single day that no matter what I am going through and no matter how bad I feel there is always something positive. Just one positive thought every day can heal your emotions over time. You're going through a lot and so much to think about.

Here are some of the emotional effects of PCOS:

DEPRESSION OVER YOUR CHANGING BODY

The biggest emotional upset with PCOS is (drum roll): our changing body image. It is understandable that many people will think the hardest emotional burden of this condition is infertility, not always. The first signs of PCOS are changes in our bodies and those are what we have to deal with first. This especially impacts younger women and teens, but is still a huge headache for middle aged and older women. We all want to feel beautiful and it is hard to deal with changes in our bodies, especially weight gain and hair growth or loss. Teenagers never want to deal with weight gain and acne and it can be downright embarrassing for them to have to talk to mom about irregular periods. PCOS sufferers can really take an emotional tumble just from symptoms alone.

Thickening middle sections and muffin tops aren't very fun to deal with either. You know they notice, but they don't often comment. You wonder what they think; you take steps to conceal it by running out and buying those spanky things and wear looser and larger clothing. It may work to conceal the changes from the outside world, but inside you feel it emotionally. I used to take a shirt, pants, or dress off the rack in the store and buy it without even trying it on. I'm sure you can sympathize with the fact that with PCOS and my changing shape, I now head to the dressing rooms only to find those slinky things just don't fit right anymore. One way to get rid of muffin tops, buy your jeans and pants one size larger. It actually looks better. Another trick is to pair pants and leggings with long tunic tops and sweaters. Find your inner goddess and delight in the comfort of loose clothing that flows with you. I love long flowing skirts these days.

Fad diets, plucking hairs, and larger clothing don't always seem to fix the way you are feeling about yourself inside. You don't know who you can talk to about it, but believe me once you do you will find that more women understand than you once thought. Many women suffer from the emotional effects of body image, regardless of the cause. And if you can't find a trusted friend that understands, at least you know that I understand. It isn't easy at first, but over time you will find a new and better you developing. New clothing styles, different colors, a fresh new hairstyle and accessories are sometimes all it takes to make you feel better inside.

One thing that I found helpful is to get up and get dressed every single day no matter how bad you are feeling. There is something uplifting about getting ready for the day that can lift your spirits and make you feel better.

THE NO BABY, NO PURPOSE FEELINGS

Infertility affects anyone and everyone with PCOS. Even if you aren't planning a family, society has ingrained in women that their purpose is to bear and have children. This is a stigma that can be very hard to overcome.

This is another situation that only others that suffer from infertility will understand. The feelings can be powerful and overcome you, but don't ever let them.

If you really do want children of your own, then the affects of PCOS can cause emotional turmoil for both you and your partner. Because your periods are irregular, you may think from month to month that you are actually pregnant only to see negative results on several pregnancy tests. Each time you feel let down, like a failure and the constant longing for a child. I felt this every month for over a year and it sent me into a depression. The only way I could shake those sad feelings, was to keep trying. I kept at it and I won the battle over infertility. Then I had other feelings of guilt when my daughter was born sick and too early because of pre-eclampsia. I still live with that very guilt to this day. The only difference is I don't let it consume me. I acknowledge the feelings and move on with my day.

Even if you are not planning on having a family and do not want children, there can still be a sense of loss. As explained to me by friends who are in this position, they sometimes feel a deep sense of regret when they are around other friends with kids. This can usually set in around the late thirties to mid-fifties when people start to think about who will take care of them when they are elderly. This is a common mid-life adjustment and the situation and feelings can be navigated with advance planning for your future.

The important thing to understand is your purpose as a woman entails so much more than giving birth. Now is the time to really find yourself and learn to love yourself for the wonderful things you do for this world. I found comfort in hobbies like; crocheting, painting, ceramics, tribal drumming, and writing poetry. We are dynamic individuals and our creativity is the best way to see all that we CAN do, instead of the things that we cannot do. I have found that it takes very little effort to make my mark on this world and it is way more than the children I bore that gives people joy. Funny jokes, a poem that hits home or something I whip up in my kitchen can bring a smile to others faces. I found self satisfaction in the little things in life. I had to stop putting motherhood as a requirement in life to end those feelings.

Realizing your true purpose of sharing your talents and all that you have to give to this world is very therapeutic in many ways. You will find yourself growing stronger when you develop an, "I CAN" attitude. Find positive mantra's and place them all over your house if you have to. I like those sticky wall postings that you can get in the home decorating section of stores. Tell yourself every day that you are special and you will begin to believe it!

Dealing With The Feelings Of Those Around You

I remember walking into work one morning. My boss was pregnant and due sometime in December. I was trying to conceive and couldn't. I took one look at her pregnant belly and her cute maternity clothes and it was all I could bear. I went straight to my office, put my head down on my desk and burst into tears It felt so unfair! It was then that I realized if motherhood was something I really wanted, I was going to need to fight for it and that meant mustering up every ounce of emotional strength that I had inside of me.

PCOS is a tough road for everyone involved. It isn't just you; your partner, your family, your friends, and even your coworkers all suffer with you in some fashion. Even if you don't mean to, you wear PCOS like a bright orange coat. Dealing with the health issues is one thing, but dealing with the emotions that go with it is sometimes very hard to contain. Some of this is hormonal and a lot of it is just the effects of having the condition period. It is exhausting both physically and emotionally. The only problem is no one seems to understand how bad you feel inside.

My partner was just about at wits end of my incessant basal temperature and cycle charting. The new diet in the house was akin to rabbit food and my moods were horrid. I wouldn't have wanted to live or work with me. We fought continuously and I never once asked him how he was feeling about things. I just assumed since he wasn't suffering from PCOS that he was fine. Wrong answer! Our relationship suffered greatly during the year and a half I was trying to get pregnant with our oldest daughter. It suffered even more after the last one was born because of the ovarian failure and my body had already started into menopause. The mood swings were horrible and I was very depressed.

My partner was suffering from PCOS right alongside me. I found out later that he, too, felt devastated with every negative pregnancy test. He woke up every morning at five a.m. with me while I took my temperature. He drove me hundreds of miles for medical tests and procedures. He stayed calm to comfort me when I couldn't take anymore. You're not alone with PCOS; your partner suffers from it too. Find time to ask how they are feeling. Share things that you have learned about PCOS. And when your pregnancy tests are negative, reach out with compassion to your partner. Understand that this emotionally can affect your partner just as much as it affects you.

If you and your partner aren't planning a family, then PCOS can be just as hard in other ways. If you suffer from high blood sugar or diabetes then your partner may be affected with worries about your health. Your mood swings may be hard for them to understand. They may also be concerned if your weight has spiraled out of control and that your health is going downhill and they may lose you. The mood swings of PCOS are some of the worst in female health. Especially later in life when hormones begin to fluctuate, you may find yourself madly in love with your partner one day and hating him the next. The best way to deal with this is to educate your partner on the effects of the hormonal swings. When you feel one coming on, let them know you aren't "feeling well." This will help avoid unnecessary hurt feelings and fights for no apparent reason.

Your family is tough to deal with too. Mostly what I dealt with is lack of understanding. Everyone goes their separate ways and we all tend to lose connection a little bit. That is normal. But I felt myself having to explain things and trying to make them understand how I felt. PCOS doesn't really run in my family and I was the only one who had it. For them, it seemed like the only thing we talked about anymore was my condition. We would get through the usual; how the kids were doing in school, how was work going and general life chit-chat and then it would immediately go to how I was feeling lately. At family gatherings, I would tend to isolate myself to a safe corner on the couch because I had nothing else to talk about with anyone. What improved my relationships with my family is talking to them about the condition and updating them on my medical appointments, medical situation, and how I was feeling. They began to understand and things got better eventually. They now even know my by moods what is going on with me. It takes time and patience for everyone, but eventually it will all come around and be positive again.

At work, your coworkers may notice a change in your moods. They may also be concerned about your health and feel sad for you if you're suffering from infertility. They may also be very confused about your reactions to a pregnant coworker. You may take more sick days or half-days for medical appointments. They may wonder why you are getting preferential treatment and jealousy may develop. You may miss quite a few days if you are going through fertility cycles. This is a good time for some "lunchroom" disclosure. Include them, educate them and help your coworkers understand what dealing with PCOS takes. You may find them more supportive than you expected. If you don't feel like sharing, have a private talk with your boss about the situation and have your boss let everyone know that you are going through something at the moment that you would rather not discuss. You cannot be discriminated against for this as it is a health condition. Many companies will tread very lightly on the "fertility" issue since they can be sued for pregnancy discrimination. It is up to you how you want to handle this part but being open with others is always the best way to deal with it.

I always found myself thinking in frustration, "I wish others could have what I have just for one day so they can see how I feel." Then I had to overcome the guilt of wishing this curse on others. Not that I truly was wishing someone would get sick, but I just needed other people around me to understand how I felt. The frustration can build up to almost intolerable levels and the only way I effectively dealt with it was to find healthy ways to vent the frustrations. People will eventually come around.

I think the best defense from all of this emotional turmoil with others is education and teaching about PCOS. Getting your hands on as much literature as possible to give to others is the key to bringing them to an understanding of the condition. One thing you need to understand is that not everyone is going to understand. Accept this fact and move on. I had to let a lot of things and people go over the years because it is not worth fighting for when you need to focus on your inner circle. You, your partner, and your family are all that matter right now. Actually, during this time the smaller your inner circle you have to deal with the better. Emotionally, you will find more strength in less numbers. This is because relationships are give and take. It is best to save all your emotional energy for yourself and those around you who really need it. You will find that those who were truly your friends will always be your friends no matter what!

So Much To Think About

PCOS is a lot on your plate. Once you realize there is something wrong and you don't completely understand it yourself, you can easily slip into a depression. There are a million thoughts running through your head and you can't seem to make sense of all of it. I actually had this happen pretty quickly. I was once a bright energetic individual and PCOS was like being cut in half. I felt like half a person, not worthy and had no idea how to get out of my rut and start fighting. I had to have a way to sort out all of these thoughts and feelings, so I started keeping a journal and started writing a plan to get my life back.

Anxiety Attacks: Hormonal Imbalances and Worries

I also suffered from horrible anxiety attacks. This seemed to be connected to the way I felt physically. On bad days that I felt tired and out of sorts, feeling bad scared me. It felt like something was horribly wrong with me and my mind would wander. The more I let my mind wander and worry about how I felt physically, the anxiety would just build up to a breaking point and before I knew it I was in a "full-blown" anxiety attack. I could be going along with my day just fine and a symptom such as severe fatigue would hit and it would stop my day dead in its tracks. I would have to pull my car over, roll down the windows, and get out and pace for five minutes before I could start driving again. The anxiety attacks began to consume me. This was probably the biggest part of the emotional toll for me, anxiety attacks are paralyzing. I later found that the hormonal changes in my endocrine system is what triggered them, but it took four years of Klonopin to bring them under control and I finally weaned off medication and learned some great behavioral therapy techniques to control them without medications. I will share these techniques with you in my book on natural therapies for PCOS. They are wonderful and the good thing is that behavioral therapy techniques are non-sedating, non-addictive, and permanent. You can use them anywhere, at any time!

YOUR EMOTIONAL RESCUE PLAN

You have to have a plan. A sound plan and you need to stick to it. It is a well-known fact that people do best with structure, routine and "to-do" lists. Organizing yourself will help you deal with the emotions as they come. You will also need organization to prevent yourself from getting overwhelmed. This will also help you keep up on doctor appointments and treatments. You can also write in reminders to give your partner, family, and friends a little needed attention too. Schedule everything that you do and you will find the whirlwind of PCOS a little easier to navigate. Lab tests and other testing will be busy at first and you wouldn't want to forget an important appointment. If you suffer from stress and anxiety, this is a lifesaver. Stress will only take you down and this is the time to find strength in yourself. Become the most organized person you ever knew and life will flow smoothly.

Start journaling your feelings right away. Keep this journal and stick to it just like you will be sticking to your basal temperature charting, your blood sugar and blood pressure checks. Your emotional health is as important as your physical health. This will help you stay strong through all the bumps in the road and help you see how strong you really are when you look back and read your journal down the road. Especially if you get anxious, you can look at your symptoms and see that hormonal changes may be what fuels how you are feeling emotionally. That only comes from knowing your cycles like the back of your own hand. Then and only then will you be able to say to yourself, "You've come a long way baby!" And then someday you may be able to help others cope, just like I am doing. Journaling is exactly how I became a PCOS survivor!

Along with your journal, you need to write out a clear plan on how you are going to deal with PCOS. From dietary changes to medical treatments to alternative options, you need to learn all that you can about your options and incorporate your plan of action. I bought a spiral bound notebook so I wouldn't lose any pages. The beginning of the journal was my plan and I put tabs on the pages to section it off. Mine looked a little bit like this:

KIMMY'S PCOS PLAN

- ▶ Fertility diet (Log foods eaten)
- ▶ Do basal temperature/ovulation symptoms chart daily!
- ▶ Write in journal daily
- ▶ Join an online support group
- ▶ Keep all doctor appointments (Write down any lab appointments)
- ▶ Check blood sugars and blood pressures often
- ▶ Stick to the fertility diet (Hard One)
- ▶ Take any medications prescribed as the doctor ordered them to be taken!
- ▶ Write down the time you took your medication and how much you took.
- ▶ Write down any medication doses and update them with each doctor visit.

I wrote up my plan in a spiral notebook which doubled as my daily journal. I dated the top of each page and wrote the above list at the top. Each day I checked off each step and then wrote my journal entries on the bottom. Keep track of depression and anxiety attacks. This way you can see the root of what is causing those changes. Once you start treatment, any new symptoms may actually be a side-effect of medication. You will also need to keep track of any medications or supplements that you are taking. This way you won't forget a dose, which is very important if you are doing fertility cycles. I know this sounds a little bit anal-retentive, but you will be surprised at how much it helps you deal with PCOS. It will give you the control back over your life, when you feel like PCOS controls you.

YOU NEED SUPPORT

"Encourage, lift and strengthen one another. For the positive energy spread will be felt by us all. For we are all connected, one and all." Deborah Day

No matter how hard to try to get people to understand PCOS, they will never completely understand. Find a PCOS support group either online or in your home community. They are out there waiting for you to join in. Experienced sufferers are a wealth of information and soon your experience is going to help someone else. It's all about networking and because of this, I got the answers and help that I needed. I am including an Appendix at the end of this book with helpful resources to find a good support group.

Many of your social networking sites have wonderful support groups built right into the sites. They are extremely confidential and often require an explanation of why you want to join (To avoid spammers of course). Once you are in, you will find a place where you can "tell all," without judgement and a world of knowledge and understanding. You can ask lots of questions and no question is a dumb question. They love to help and teach in most of these groups. Now remember your doctor is the expert and be very wary of people trying to practice medicine. There are some dangerous practices out there so use good judgement. Any questions regarding medications and lab results need to be answered by your doctor. I did find that support groups make some pretty good suggestions to steer you in the right direction with the right questions to ask your doctor.

Your local hospital may have a referral service for support groups that meet locally in your community. This tends to bring things closer to home and you may make some new friends that you can get together with and meet with outside of group. Hospital support groups are often run by trained staff that understands what you are going through, as well as PCOS survivors in your community. It is important to believe who you are talking to about your condition when you're looking for understanding.

If you do see a fertility specialist or enter into a fertility/IVF program, they will most likely refer you to and highly encourage you to meet up with some of their other patients for support. Fertility specialists like it when their patients connect with each other and the support groups are run by people who are trained to understand what you are going through as well as former fertility patients to help see you through this time. I also highly recommend these types of groups. My obstetrician with my oldest daughter recommended a group connected with his practice and I don't know what I would have done without that weekly meeting during the time we were conceiving and throughout my pregnancy. It was fun and gave us a chance to mingle with others who understood what we were going through.

The good thing about our support group was once I became pregnant we transferred over to the "high risk" pregnancy group and I had others to share with while I was going through complications during pregnancy. It also separates you from the people who are still going through fertility treatments to avoid hard feelings. I even had a "parents of preemies" support group that was amazing after my daughter was born early due to my pre-eclampsia. They helped me understand what was going on and get over the feelings of guilt I had because my baby was sick.

I am such a big proponent of support groups and even have a few different ones today that address different sides of my autoimmune condition. They have so much information that is useful and are there with a kind shoulder when I feel down. I don't know what I would do without them. From doctor referrals to side-effects of medications that we all share, it is a priceless blessing to have people that understand what you are going through.

Here are a few helpful tips when choosing a support group:

Take your time and do your research. You can scope out online groups and local support groups to get a "feel" how they work. There are certain qualities that you need to look for in groups.

Ask yourself what you expect. In order for a support group to be helpful, you need to understand why you yourself are there in the first place. This way you can identify faster if the group will be able to fulfill your needs.

Look for a warm, caring and compassionate environment. Watch out for unnecessary venting, flaming, and control issues. Choose an environment that is well moderated with people who have a mutual respect for one another. With online groups, you usually have to read an agreement disapproving of such behavior and need to be approved before you join. Go through the online forums and read some of the messages. When you visit a physical group, go a few times and watch that each person is given time to have the "floor" and that the group administrator knows how to balance this.

Community and outreach is important. Look for a group that personally welcomes new members. There should also be an outreach team that can help you in times of crisis or need. It is also helpful to have outings and meet-ups for people to forge solid relationships with one another.

Know when it is time to move on. If a group is not fulfilling your needs, it is acceptable to move on. There are plenty of groups out there and if you have exhausted efforts with physical groups move to an online support group.

No matter what kind of support group you choose for yourself, any kind of support will help you during this time. Take your partner along or include them in your online groups. They need support too and it may help them see that you are not alone with your symptoms.

COMING TO TERMS WITH PCOS

Once you have been positively diagnosed, PCOS is just going to become a part of your daily life. At first you will be overwhelmed with what you have to do to be healthy again. In time, you will learn to deal with it. If you find yourself worrying about things from day to day, write down the phrase I used at the beginning of this chapter. PCOS is something you can control, but never let it control you. It is very easy to get caught up in an illness. PCOS affects your overall physical and emotional state and at first, it may be all that you think about. You may find yourself letting go of some of the very things you once loved to do. Don't do that. Try to live as normally as possible. Keep up with your hobbies, social life, and think of the future. Make plans and don't break them. You will find with PCOS that the more you do for yourself, the better you will start to feel.

You will soon find that checking temperatures, blood sugars, blood pressures, and taking medications are just a daily routine. At first it will feel like a chore. Sex may feel like a scheduled activity, so find ways to make it feel spontaneous. Your diet may get old and boring, so find healthy ways to spice that up a little too. There are some excellent cookbooks out there tailored for diabetics and PCOS sufferers that fit into your lifestyle very well and taste great! But don't let this be all you do for yourself. Make those things part of your daily routine, like brushing your teeth. Set aside time for yourself in the evenings to do something you like to do. I wrote some great poetry and crocheted many a blanket. I was surprised how much things like that cleared my mind and refreshed me for the next day. I even sat and made myself complete a one thousand piece jigsaw puzzles. Whatever I could find that kept my mind off of my illness. I think the worst times for me were those times closest to my expected period when I was trying to conceive. That was when I had the most nervous energy. I wanted to see if the pregnancy tests would be positive even before my missed periods. I spent a lot of money that I could have used for other things that benefited my emotional health more. Like getting my nails or hair done and feeling better about myself.

Once you get skilled at journaling, you will find your feelings kind of "stick" to the journal pages and don't haunt you as much. Over time you won't even wake up thinking about it. But, it is about having a good routine and schedule. When I have too much time on my hands, I start to think about it again. Then I start to feel the physical and emotional effects again. Keep up with your hobbies and your social life as much as you can. I cannot stress the importance of that enough. If you find yourself out and the social anxiety or withdrawal sets in, take a break for only a minute and get right back at it. If you see a pregnant woman and start to cry, leave the room and get control of those feelings. If you see people healthy and happy, realize that you are healthy and happy too. With PCOS, you are no different from anyone else really. You have to keep telling yourself that. I realized that no amount of bed rest made it go away and getting out and about didn't kill me either. It was just something I had to overcome and come to terms with.

Having a baby won't fix it either. I found that out the hard way. As soon as the pregnancy hormones wore off, I felt terrible again. It took about a year or two after each pregnancy and then I was right back at square one. After having three of my four children with PCOS, I have found that it still exists and the only thing that satisfied me was turning the "sufferer" into a "survivor" title. With education comes understanding and with understanding comes acceptance and only in that order. The only way I found to deal with all of the feelings, was to confront them head-on each time they surfaced. Understand that the bad days do go away.

Most of my bad days were riddled with anxiety attacks. Not only is this an emotional response, but also a physical one. Your endocrine system is connected to your nervous system. This is how the body communicates what it needs and where. When a hormone is off, your adrenal glands kick in to help your body to keep going temporarily. Over time, your panic button gets stuck in the on position and you can possibly develop full-blown Generalized Anxiety Disorder. This happened to me and I had to seek treatment for that too. I was only on anxiety medications for a short time and then I learned to control the attacks with cognitive behavioral techniques. When my hormones stabilized, the attacks finally left me just as quickly as they started. They were terrifying to live with and there were days I never left the house for fear of having an attack. Somehow, I learned to cope and the anxiety and other emotions became easier to deal with. You will learn to cope too.

PCOS is like the changing seasons. As I sit here and write this book looking at the snowflakes falling outside my window, I think back to the seasons of PCOS. At first, I weathered the hard cold winter. It was the unknown darkness I feared, until I found the needed tools to learn. When understanding came, so did the spring. I felt like I blossomed for the very first time in my life. Not only did I give birth to children but also to a new me. I frolicked in the happiness and health of my new life in the summertime, only to find that in the fall I started to withdraw back into the darkness. I have lived through so many seasons of PCOS, but the good thing is, I now know what to expect when the changes come. The symptoms are pretty much the same with every cycle, just like the changing seasons. This is why journaling your symptoms is so very important. You are literally getting to know yourself and that is often something we forget to do.

To sum it all up, you need to understand that PCOS is a part of your life and somehow with good planning, education, and a little work you can make it fit in. You will benefit much better in the long-run to not fight it, but instead "roll with the punches." Before you know it, you won't think in terms of PCOS sufferer, you will be a PCOS survivor!

Chapter Four

The PCOS Diagnosis

"Diagnosis is not the end, but the beginning of practice."
– Martin H. Fischer

I knew something wasn't right. I tend to trust my gut feelings more than anything. I doctor hopped for quite some time and was brushed off. I took it into my own hands and began to research my symptoms. Now, at the time internet wasn't that popular and I didn't even know what an e-mail address was. I was starting my journey into researching what I had in the middle of the 1990s and at the time didn't even own a computer. I don't quite remember how I found my information on PCOS, but I do know that it was in book format. I wasn't positively diagnosed yet, but I decided to start some sound health practices that were geared toward people with PCOS.

My husband and I had been married for almost a year and decided we wanted a baby. I wasn't using birth control and wasn't getting pregnant. I had other symptoms too. Noticeable hairs on my chin and my chest, period cycles of thirty-seven days instead of twenty-eight and I was extremely thin. One of the first things I read was that super thin girls do not have enough estrogen to induce ovulation. I was also athletic and thought that because I worked out so much, I had somehow increased my body's testosterone.

At this time, I didn't know I had PCOS, but I surely suspected it. So, I picked up a book on diet to help balance my fluctuating weight, balance my hormones, and increase chances of fertility.

I started the diet and it truly was "rabbit food." I had to increase my intake of B vitamins, whole grains and decrease caffeine, simple carbohydrates and junk food. It wasn't very pleasant for me or my husband, since we were busy and it was hard to cook properly. The diet consists of a lot of leafy greens, so we learned to make fun dinner salads paired with lean protein meats. It was using the PCOS diet that actually tipped me off that I might have PCOS, only because I became pregnant with our first child pretty quickly on the diet and using basal charting.

I still lived with only suspicion, because denial on my part and being brushed off by physicians only delayed my diagnosis. I was actually a very healthy person and my basic lab tests looked great all the time. There was nothing there to tip off any of my regular doctors. Of course, my obstetrician didn't think there was a problem at this point because he had run basic tests on both me and my husband during our fertility work-up. Everything looked fine and I got pregnant. It was just the luck of the draw, the diet and a lot of hard work. The medical attention stopped there and when I developed pre-eclampsia my doctor wasn't really inclined to look into any reasons why, he just treated it and we moved on. In hindsight, I see it as another missed clue. Still, I wrote down all of these clues in my spiral notebook and when I filled up one book, I placed it in a box and started another.

It wasn't until after my last child was born that all of the symptoms seemed to lead somewhere and it was actually a doctor that I worked with in the hospital as a nurse who noticed what my symptoms pointed to. Not everyone has the chance to work so closely with a doctor on a daily basis, but he saw the signs. He was the one who referred me to the reproductive endocrinologist that would solve the mystery. I couldn't have been any more persistent with the previous doctor's-- they just don't have the time. So, in my case it was a blessing that someone finally noticed that something was not quite right with me. It was then that I dug through all of my boxes of keepsakes and found my journals. Then the work began. I made a detailed list of all of my symptoms and health issues over the last ten years. When I was finished, I had a pretty clear picture to show the endocrinologist. I was ready to go!

If you suspect that you might have PCOS, your first step is to research it as much as you can. Remember that a lot of conditions can mimic PCOS and PCOS can mimic other conditions. If you have symptoms of high blood sugar, high blood pressure and irregular periods, it does warrant a good thorough physical from your physician. High blood sugar and blood pressure are nothing to play around with and need to be addressed as soon as possible. Once you have that out of the way, it is time to get to work on getting your referral. If your doctor finds even a borderline high blood sugar and your gaining weight, it might be a good idea to bring up the suggestion of PCOS. If you have already been charting your basal temperatures and monthly cycles and this will help your case even more, don't ever let your doctor tell you that forty-two day cycles are normal. They are not. Try not to let them be too quick to try and put you on birth control to "regulate" your cycles either. Ask them if you can have a full work-up by a reproductive endocrinologist before you start any form of treatment.

Most importantly, try not to doctor hop. I realize now that I made a huge mistake in doing that. One doctor needs to keep seeing you. Even if they shove you off and tell you nothing is wrong at first or even over a period of time. You need to keep at it and report any new symptoms.

Every time you start a new relationship with a new doctor, you will have to start all over again. They will need to take a thorough history; physical, initial lab tests and these may show that nothing is wrong. Remember, one doctor may have hundreds of patients to manage and they need time to get to know you and your body. Doctors that seem to brush you off may take note of your symptoms and actually be thinking about how they fit in. Be patient.

If you truly do have a doctor that really does seem to be dismissing your complaints, then maybe it is time to find a new doctor. Just think through this carefully and check into your physicians when looking for a new doctor. You can always ask the receptionist when calling if the doctor takes an interest in PCOS and endocrine disease. Keep looking until you find one. Also, some doctors list areas of interest on their physician profiles on the internet. You may even find that you have to commute to a different city, but doing that may be worth the trip.

SEEING THE REPRODUCTIVE ENDOCRINOLOGIST

Once you get into a reproductive endocrinologist, they will take a thorough history and ask for your symptoms. This is when you get to hand them you're well drawn up list based on your journaling. Having the list compiled will save time for them, since they may not want to flip through all of your journals. They will also ask for any medications you are currently on. Your average menstrual cycle length and if you have been trying to get pregnant.

Then they may order the following tests including:

- Insulin Level
- Glucose Level
- Hemoglobin A1C (Checks average of blood sugar over 3 months)
- Luteinizing Hormone
- Follicle Stimulating Hormone
- Testosterone
- Androstenedione
- Estrogen Level
- Cholesterol/Lipids
- DHEA
- Prolactin
- Cortisol Levels
- Other tests as deemed necessary by your endocrinologist (i.e. fasting leptin, SHBG, etcetera)

Understand that there isn't one set test that can actually diagnose PCOS. The diagnosis is actually made by meeting certain criteria, along with elevated levels of certain hormones. There may not be any elevation in hormone levels, but the weight gain, infertility and excess hair growth are obvious.

When I had my testing done, the reproductive endocrinologist did them in the office, first thing in the morning by intravenous blood draw. Androgens and steroids can become elevated under stress. The doctor had me come in fasting, first thing in the morning and started an IV. She then had me go into the waiting room and read a magazine for fifteen minutes. This helps stabilize the hormones that may rise due to the stress of driving to the office and having a needle inserted in your arm. If you experience panic or anxiety, it may be a good idea to ask your doctor if they test in this fashion.

Remember to let your doctor know when your last period was and keep track of them if they are very irregular. Some hormones are best tested at certain times. If everything comes back normal the first time, do not hesitate to ask to be re-tested if your insurance will allow it. Be persistent!

CRITERIA FOR PCOS DIAGNOSIS

The criteria for diagnosis of PCOS have been set by three different health agencies for use by physicians. You may be asked questions about your symptoms and the doctor may make some physical observations. The criteria based diagnosis is only made after the doctor rules out any other causes for your symptoms. Here are the criteria for the diagnosis of PCOS:

NATIONAL INSTITUTES OF HEALTH (NIH) NEEDS ALL THREE OF THE FOLLOWING:

1. Must have clinical or biochemical evidence of hyperandrogenism (elevated levels on lab testing)

2. Oligomenorrhea and/or anovulation (Cycles over 35 days/No ovulation)

3. Other conditions have been excluded as the cause of symptoms

In explanation of number 3, when you first go to your personal physician you most likely will have a battery of lab tests. They often come back normal and this is the reason people doctor hop. When you have true PCOS, usually your organs are all working fine. Your blood counts are normal, your liver is normal, and your kidneys are normal. But, it is important to exclude any other possible causes for your symptoms before you can go on to a full PCOS work-up. And once again, try not to doctor hop. This only breaks up the pieces of the puzzle and you will be lucky to find a doctor that can put it all back together again. I may have had my diagnosis a lot sooner if I had stuck it out with one doctor. Mood swings and heightened emotions may make you frustrated, but one person needs to see the whole picture. That is your personal physician. Stay with them long enough to get to know you.

When the diagnosis is made, only a trained eye can spot the signs of PCOS. This is why at least one visit with a medical doctor is important to make sure the right tests are run. If you do have blood sugar or blood pressure problems, you may need to be monitored by your physician and obtain treatment until the levels stabilize. This is very important. Blood sugar and blood pressure needs to be stabilized and monitored. After my last pregnancy, my blood pressure was 190/110 and I needed to be on blood pressure medications. During the pregnancy, I had gestational diabetes with blood sugar levels at almost 200mg/dl. I needed to be on insulin shots during the pregnancy and now I just follow the PCOS diet and haven't had any other problems since. After some time I was able to stop taking it and remained normal, but I still had it checked just to be on the safe side. I still have my blood sugar checked every few months randomly, as well.

By now, you're most certainly wrapped up in the whirlwind of PCOS. You're being spun in every direction and you're unsure of how to keep it all together. Keep up with your plan, your journal, and your list every day. Once the lab testing and work-up appointments are out of the way, it should be pretty clear sailing. Like the quote at the beginning of this section, now it is time to put everything into practice!

After diagnosis, you will be faced with one tough situation if you are trying to have a baby. The financial impact of fertility treatments can be just as rough as your symptoms. It may even affect you more than the anxiety and depression, or it can add to the emotional impact.

PCOS Diagnosis and The Financial Impact

Well, what can I say? I am glad that when I was diagnosed I had health insurance to pay for the lab testing. Some of the lab tests done for PCOS are very common every day tests. When you get into the specialized endocrine testing, it can run into the thousands of dollars. Make sure to check with your reproductive endocrinologist on which tests will be run and check with your insurance to make sure they are covered before they are performed. This way, there are no surprises. Chances are the androgen testing will be covered and fertility testing may not be.

The medical aspect of PCOS is covered. You can receive diabetic testing supplies, medications, and associated doctor visits. The fertility part is the tricky one. Most insurance policies do not cover the cost of fertility treatments or they cover very little. More and more insurances are beginning to cover more fertility treatment costs, but it is slow going. If you have no health insurance it would be a good idea to get on a small plan prior to diagnosis. You wouldn't want to be stuck needing medications or treatments that you cannot afford.

The out-of-pocket costs on fertility treatment can run into the thousands per cycle. Drugs to induce ovulation average about $1,000 to $3,000 per cycle. IVF averages up to $10,000 per cycle. There are programs out there where you can receive large discounts on treatment and you may receive a full refund of the fees if you are unsuccessful getting pregnant. Fertility programs also have financing available to help you make payments on the costs, instead of coming up with a lump sum payment. I am including links to some of these programs in the Appendix at the end of this book.

I can honestly say that some people want babies so badly, they sell their home and cars. They go through numerous cycles and are defeated each time. Only to find when they gave up completely, they ended up pregnant.

But when you want a baby so badly, you would give up anything and everything just to have one. So, there are programs out there to help relieve that financial burden and I highly recommend you contact them. It is also a good idea to contact the programs early on after diagnosis, since the application phase can take some time. They also have financial counselors available to help you with budgeting in your treatments. Just finding the help and the answers you need helps to ease at least one of the burdens of PCOS. Financial strain can really contribute to strife with your partner. Don't let it, get help as soon as you know you have this.

The financial impact of PCOS is the reason why some people choose not to have children. The good news here is that some of the treatments for the medical portion of PCOS help to treat the infertility and then there are no extra out-of-pocket expenses. For instance, metformin helps to increase the body's sensitivity to insulin, reduce androgen levels and in many women induces successful ovulation. I know, I was one of them. I had no intentions of having a baby at thirty-eight years old, but my endocrinologist forgot to tell me the one side-effect that made that happen and, viola, I have my youngest daughter. A beautiful surprise, no doubt! Even just the diet, weight loss, and exercise portion of treatments can successfully induce ovulation and help to regulate periods. It just takes finding what is going to work for your body. It may be less expensive that you thought it was going to be.

Financial planning for PCOS and infertility will give you an idea of what you have to spend. Knowing up front what you are looking at will help you create a livable budget. Yes, you may have to cut out a few eating out or coffee sessions every week, but you will surprise yourself at how much you really can save. And anything you can get your insurance to cover under the "medical necessity" umbrella will really help. There are more treatments out there that have dual purpose than you know and even if something gets denied by insurance; your doctor can help you write an appeal letter to prove medical necessity. Many companies that sponsor health insurance can also help appeal certain provisions on the policy and it has been done for PCOS and infertility. It is worth trying for!

Chapter Five

Positively PCOS, Now What?

"The news comes somewhat late, but I am glad to hear it nevertheless" Malcolm Campbell

It was an unforgettable day at my doctor's office. The words rang out so clearly, like church bells in the vicinity. "I am 99.9 percent sure you have PCOS," she told me.

"Are you sure," I asked?

"Yes, the labs are showing elevations in your androgens. You also have hyperglycemia and your blood pressures are pretty high," she answered. I don't know why I questioned her as I should have been jumping for joy that someone finally figured out what was wrong with me. I already knew myself this was probably what I had, but hearing the sureness in my doctor's voice was no less comforting than having a lead brick dropped on your toes. Total Shock!

Shocking to know I had PCOS, but also a sense of relief that a doctor had finally found what was making me sick all these years. It was these first feelings of shock that were the hardest to deal with. I was miserable for years prior, had trouble getting pregnant, sick during my pregnancies and just completely brushed off by the medical community. I felt anger for my suffering, I felt relief that I was going to get help, I felt bad for my husband

and all that he went through, and I was so confused. I had a lot of questions like, "will the treatment work," "will I have side-effects," and "will I need to take insulin shots," I asked my doctor? She reassured me that usually the most minor treatments for PCOS are very successful. Metformin is the mainstay and first line of treatment and the majority of people have very good luck with it, there is a moderately high pregnancy success rate in those who use Metformin. Still, I was worried because I knew it had side-effects and wondered if it would drop my blood sugar too low.

The first thing I did was look up the medication I was going to be taking, but I still took it like the doctor told me to. I also checked my blood sugar and blood pressure on a regular basis. I logged my blood sugars and I went on a sugar-free diet. I started to look at the condition as a door to better health, instead of a sentence to illness. I took on a whole new outlook on life and there was no stopping me. It was ten-plus years after I used journaling and charting for fertility, I was now going to use the same plan for managing my condition. I was ready to make a new plan and stick with it for my health.

I think it was the shock of finding out my diagnosis that helped me build the most strength towards getting healthy. To me the "bad news" was actually good news, because I was finally going to get help for my condition. I was finally going to have a life again!

TIME TO TALK TO YOUR LOVED ONES ABOUT PCOS

After I gathered my feelings and developed my new outlook, it did take a little time before I was ready tell my partner, family, and friends about my diagnosis. To tell you the truth, they weren't that shocked or interested, for that matter. It didn't seem like as big a deal to them as it was to me. Then again, others don't really understand the full impact of PCOS unless they suffer from it. Don't expect people to jump for joy for you or throw a party. Once you break the news, it's pretty much going to be "business as usual." That is okay. This is why signing up for a PCOS support group is so very important. These are the people who will give you the needed "pats on the back" and cheer you on every step of your journey with PCOS. They will also help you once you begin your treatment and help you understand how the medications and treatment will make you feel. Your support group will understand everything first hand. You may be a little shy with it at first, just remember you need the support of your loved ones.

Don't hold back. It is soon going to be time to tell your partner, family, friends, and your coworkers what has been going on with you. Along with knowing your diagnosis, give them the education they need to understand what you are going through. You will soon discover they are more interested than you once thought. People often don't talk about things or offer support, because they just don't understand. Be prepared to answer questions. They will want to know if you are sick. They will want to know if you can have children. They will slowly come out of their own shock and open back up to you.

At work, your boss may cut you some slack for doctor and lab appointments. These are going to be important to keep. Your coworkers will be a little less mortified when you pull out the glucose monitor at the lunch table and a little less offended when you turn down that decadent cake made for your coworkers birthday. Get them in on it too. You can have lunchtime weigh-ins and encourage each other if some want to join in on losing weight or eating better. Encourage healthy eating at office potlucks and bring in fruit trays for desserts. You can integrate this into your career life. When I was at work after PCOS, we started ordering healthy turkey subs and light pasta salads that we all seemed to crave after a while. Gone were the burgers, fries, and burritos and we all enjoyed the new fare together. Fruit trays quickly overcame cakes for birthdays and we all enjoyed the weigh-ins and celebrated our victories together.

Your partner will ease into your new routine with you and maybe even help to remind you to take your medications. You may even start to find yourselves bonding closer and closer through all of this. Some partners and families may detest the new diet but, as I said before, there are wonderful cookbooks that make the diet taste really good. It is actually not even a diet, just watching the foods that tend to spike your blood sugar faster.

There is nothing against you eating a bowl or two of ice cream a week. Just remember to keep your partners feelings in mind and allow them to talk to you about themselves once in a while.

You may find your partner needs a little time to digest your diagnosis. This will pass and they will be ready to talk about it in time. Be ready to answer questions and include them in your doctor visits. If you find good points or positive quotes in this book, read it to them. This book was written with everyone in mind. Always remember they need support too.

Another very important reason for others to know is if you are put on an anti-diabetic medication you will need people to understand the symptoms of low-blood sugar. Your blood sugars can drop seriously low and rapidly. Others who are around you will need to know what to do if this happens and if they do not know you are being treated, you could end up with a very serious situation. Even if you don't tell them everything, educate them on what you are taking and the symptoms of low-blood sugar. Let them know where you keep your glucose monitor and rescue glucose, just to be safe.

Over time, people will come around and talk to you more about your condition. Just be prepared for questions and know the right answers.

DECIDE YOUR COURSE OF ACTION

If you are having problems with your blood sugar, your doctor may put you on an oral anti-diabetic agent to help control blood sugar. There is an added benefit, these drugs also help lower the production and release of androgens and can help the ovary release eggs. The risk of using this medication is hypoglycemia, or causing your blood sugar to drop too low. You will need to carry your glucose monitor, a source of quick glucose to eat and never skip meals or snacks. Another option the doctor may suggest is putting you on birth control pills, which will prevent pregnancy but give the ovaries a "rest." The decision will be up to you and how severe your case is. It is also very dangerous to use hormones if you smoke and if you are over thirty-five. There is an increased risk of blood clots with birth control pills and you need to outweigh the benefits vs. the risks if this is the route you choose to take. Hormones are not usually the first line of treatment, but can be helpful to regulate periods in younger PCOS sufferers.

Prior to my actual medical diagnosis of PCOS, I was able to conceive and give birth to two beautiful babies. I did this with a fertility diet that helps to lower blood sugar naturally and balance the body's hormones. I also used the basal temperature and cervical mucus charting method. This worked for me and I realized after my diagnosis was made that a number or combination of treatments can be combined to effectively treat the condition and increase fertility. It is pretty much up to your personal preference. It takes a lot of work, but it is so worth it and very cost-effective. Be prepared to take your temperature and chart as soon as you open your eyes in the morning.

The natural craze is growing rapidly. Everyone is looking at the effect that synthetic medications, chemicals in food and in our air has on our bodies. We are getting more and more health conscious and back to the basics. With PCOS, the decision on how you wish to treat it is entirely up to you. My advice as a nurse; however, is that any medical manifestations like high blood sugars need to be closely monitored by a physician and treated properly per the doctor's orders. This will avoid later complications such as kidney failure, heart disease, and organ and nerve damage. If you need to be on diabetic medications, please do not hesitate. But if your doctor gives you the "go-ahead" to manage your condition with diet, by all means please do!

I also believe in a combination of diet, yoga, meditation, and medications if needed. I think combining Western medicine with Natural Holistic approaches can be a very effective way to treat PCOS and good for your body. In my companion books, I will be outlining these very methods and a diet that really works. Just remember, go over your alternative choices with your doctor if you decide to do this route. Especially if you are using any herbal supplements to avoid any interactions or unwanted side-effects.

Look at all your options carefully and go over them with your partner.

Include your partner in your treatment decisions. Let them know all of the side-effects, drug interactions, and success rates. Don't hold back with anything so there are no surprises. If you need to take an anti-diabetic such as Metformin, you need to let them know what to do if you blood sugar drops too low. Also, the success rates of pregnancy with this drug. You will want to make sure you and your partner are both ready for the successes of treatment and the complications if any should arise.

WHAT ARE THE TREATMENT OPTIONS FOR PCOS?

PCOS is treated based on what part of the body is affected and if you are trying to conceive. In my case, I wasn't trying to conceive after diagnosis, but it happened. Surprise! I based my treatment regimen on a combination of both western medicine and alternative medicine. I had to do what worked for me. There are so many proponents of either one or the other out there. It isn't my job to sway you to either side; my job is to inform you of all of your options. There are some that say the "all-natural" approach is the way to go and some that will insist on Western medicine, doctors and medications. Do your research, talk to your doctor, and see what you can do to stay as healthy as possible, but feel comfortable with the treatment program you have chosen.

Whatever treatment plan you decide on, stick with it. See your doctor for lab tests regularly. Check your blood sugars, your blood pressures, and use birth control if necessary. Make sure that you inform your doctor of any other treatments you decide to use in conjunction with prescription medications for safety. The decision is entirely up to you on how you want to treat your PCOS, just remember high blood pressure and high blood sugars can be dangerous and should be carefully monitored to prevent complications.

Let's go over some of the treatment options.

WESTERN MEDICINE

High-Fiber, High-Protein and Low Glycemic Diet It is always best to try a change in diet before anything else. Doctors usually recommend trying this route first to see if your body responds and corrects the condition itself and this is entirely possible. You can do this yourself at home and there are many PCOS diet plans to fit your lifestyle without having to sacrifice flavor and fun! Watch for my own PCOS diet in the companion book to this one.

A diet for successful fertility and better blood sugar control needs to be balanced and contain essential vitamins and minerals. Even if you end up needing any of the below medications, proper diet will help keep you at your best health. It is also important to remember to eat. Starving your body is not healthy, will not help you keep off lost weight and could be dangerous if you are using medications to control blood sugar. Your body needs at least three meals a day and two to three snacks. Another way to do this is eat six small meals a day. This helps to keep steady blood sugar levels and that is very important with PCOS. It will also help your body balance androgens naturally. Losing as little as ten pounds can help your body start turning around in a positive direction.

Your physician can refer you to a licensed dietician that will design a diet plan for your needs. Again, ask about qualifications and knowledge of PCOS when visiting a dietician. Most often, the same diet used for diabetics will work well for PCOS with the addition of B vitamin containing foods and foods rich in Omega-3 fatty acids. The diet is not actually a "weight-loss" diet, unless you are overweight. Your calorie intake should remain at a healthy 1500 to 2000 calorie a day diet; you will just be eating less fat and carbohydrate calories. The trick is to increase exercise above your caloric intake. You will need to burn more than you take in.

You have to learn to like and drink water. Your body needs it and it helps flush out glucose if your blood sugars get too high. It also helps to flush out toxins. This is an important point with any dietary changes. You have to drink plenty of water. I never liked water, but paid dearly for drinking packaged drink mixes and soda. My kidneys began to fail during my second pregnancy. I quickly learned to drink more water and they got better after I cut out processed beverages.

Anti-Diabetic Medications These help increase your body's response to insulin. This helps to control out of whack blood sugars and reduces androgen production. If you don't want to become pregnant, you may need to use birth control. The reduction of androgens causes mature egg follicles to be released and you may become pregnant. Quickly!

Some women who do not respond from just one anti-diabetic medication do very well on a combination therapy of two different anti-diabetics. This combination therapy is commonly used for Type 2 Diabetes and works well for PCOS. If you find yourself prescribed these types of medications, it is going to be extremely important to check your blood sugars at least twice daily and understand the symptoms of low blood sugar. You will need to carry a glucose monitor and know what to do to bring your blood sugar up if it drops. Always carry some form of full sugar candy in your pocket or purse. I cannot stress enough that this is where you need to tell others what you are taking and what you are taking it for. Educate them on the symptoms of low-blood sugar and tell them where your rescue glucose is. Low-blood sugar can usually be caught early enough, but you will want others to know how to help you if you need it.

Side-effects of these medications include; diarrhea, interactions with alcohol, muscle pain, swelling, gas, and hypoglycemia (low-blood sugar).

Anti-Androgen Medications These are used with birth control pills to help lower the production of androgens in females. One of the most commonly used medications is spironolactone. It has been shown to help control excess hair growth in women. This is a diuretic and blood pressure medication. It is a good idea to have a blood pressure monitor at home and know the signs of low blood pressure. If you do not have kidney disease, make sure you drink plenty of fluids with this medication to avoid dehydration. Check your blood pressure in the morning before taking it and ask your doctor for parameters when the medication should be held, for instance if your blood pressure is less than 100/60. Those parameters are up to your doctor, but you would not want to take a pill that lowers blood pressure if your blood pressure is too low. This is another reason to inform loved ones and coworkers what you are taking and what for.

Side-effects of these medications include; drowsiness, headaches, nausea, diarrhea, liver problems, and irregular periods.

Oral Contraception Sometimes just regulating menstrual cycles can bring things back under control. These are given based on the thought that extra estrogen and progesterone will lower the androgens in the body. There is a brand of contraceptives that contains spironolactone and hormones that is marketed specifically for PCOS sufferers. The reviews on this drug are 50/50. Some people love it and some people are dead-set against it after experiencing severe side-effects. Just remember to do your drug research before trying anything. Always make informed choices. Also, this method will prevent you from becoming pregnant and not always the best option if you are trying to have a baby. Your doctor may want to "rest" your ovaries and stabilize your hormones before trying to become pregnant. If this is the case, you may find it very easy to become pregnant after stopping "the pill".

Know that oral contraception does have risks of its own. If you are a smoker, over thirty-five, or both, you are at increased risk of blood clots. There can be serious implications with this and you need to make yourself aware of that. The birth control method of treatment is almost always only used in younger women and teenagers to help regulate periods. Even this group needs to be aware of the risks, although they are lower in younger women.

Side-effects of these medications include; morning sickness, appetite loss, breast tenderness and pain, blood clots, spotting, hair loss, mood swings, and headaches.

Fertility Medications If you want to have a baby and there is no response to Metformin, the doctor may try adding Clomid after a few months. Clomid is a fertility drug that induces ovulation. This drug is taken during the first few days of the cycle and then a method is used to detect mature follicles. You will most likely use an ovulation predictor test or go in for an ultrasound around mid-cycle. This medication is also very effective when used in combination with anti-diabetic medications. With this treatment, the risk for multiple births is higher because several follicles release eggs at the same time. There are other types of fertility medications that I will go into detail on later.

Clomid does not have a very high success rate when used by itself. The odds of becoming pregnant on Clomid alone are about 30 percent. That isn't too bad considering a healthy woman with no medical issues only has about a 25 percent chance of getting pregnant. There are many women that have had success with Clomid. Success rates climb dramatically when used with Metformin.

Do your research on fertility drugs. Cycles can be expensive and you want to make sure they will work. Ask your doctor plenty of questions and always try the natural way first. It takes at least a year to get pregnant naturally, so give it time before you dive into these methods.

Side-effects of these medications include; abdominal pain, hot flashes, over-stimulated ovaries, hair loss, possible ovarian tumors, dizzy spells, and increased fatigue.

Surgical Intervention A laparoscopy can be performed and the surgeon can make small incisions into the follicles and cause the eggs to release. **(See Figure 6)** This technique also helps to lower excess androgens. Tumors that secrete androgens can be removed during the process and with this treatment; most women that have it can get pregnant very successfully on their own.

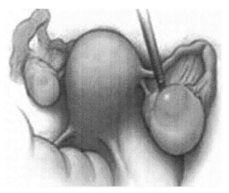

Figure 6: Ovarian Drilling
Photo Courtesy of: nezhat.org

In Vitro Fertilization (IVF) As a last resort for conception, a fertility specialist can fertilize several eggs in the laboratory and then place them back in the uterus for implantation. Anywhere from five to ten embryos are created at a time. The only setback is the incidence for multiple births is very high. There is also a higher rate of miscarriage in some women and the pregnancy needs to be monitored carefully by a specialist. IVF can range in the tens of thousands of dollars.

For severe cases of PCOS, where the egg follicles never mature, donor eggs can be used. This has been very successful in older women wanting children. Donor eggs will cause the IVF cycle costs to go up considerably as you will have to pay for the donor's medical care and medications for the cycles.

With IVF, you will also be placed on hormones to increase ovulation and regulate your cycles for optimal egg retrieval. Those follicles will need to be mature and healthy!

High Blood Pressure Medications Unrelated to fertility, you may need to be put on medication to lower your blood pressure. Hypertension is blood pressure that is higher than 120/80. They did find in my case that hypertension was transient and temporary and, after I was treated, my blood pressure returned to normal. Blood pressure medications that work best for PCOS sufferers are actually medications that affect blood pressure via the kidneys.

Side-effects of these medications include; dizziness, headaches, increased urination, "asthma like" coughing spells, rashes, and itching.

Cholesterol Lowering Drugs You may have higher cholesterol levels with PCOS and you may need to be put on cholesterol lowering drugs for a period of time. The doctor will also suggest a change in diet. This is very important to adhere to. You will need to lower your total cholesterol, low density lipoproteins, and triglycerides while raising your high density lipoproteins with "good fats" and Omega 3 fatty acids. Sometimes this can also be done with diet alone, so get on track with your diet plan as soon as possible. Again, this is always better to do naturally as cholesterol lowering medications can have side effects.

Side-effects of these medications include; stomach pain, nausea, constipation, bloating, gas, muscle pain, and fatigue.

Doctors will always tell you that with side-effects the benefits of the medication always outweighs the risks of not taking it if you need it. Research your medications and take them properly. If you do experience any severe side-effects then you need to contact you physician to make any changes in your routine.

ALTERNATIVE MEDICINE

The good news about Alternative medical approaches is that most of these therapies can be combined with Western medical approaches for successful treatment. The only exception is if you choose to use herbal therapies you will need to let your doctor know anything and everything you are taking at home to avoid any nasty drug interactions. You would never want to add to the misery of PCOS by taking your medications wrong. Some herbs can mimic the effects of synthetic drugs such as Mexican Wild Yam (Progesterone) and Soy (Estrogens).

Yoga can help during PCOS to help balance the mind and the body connection. It is a great form of exercise and I practice it regularly. The right yoga poses can help your body balance hormone levels and balance blood sugar and insulin levels. It is exercise, so it does contribute to weight loss and increasing muscle tone. You just need to take it slow when starting yoga. I will outline the best poses (asanas) in my companion book for alternative medicine.

Acupuncture is a popular form of Eastern medicine based on the theory that the body is made up of energy channels. When these channels are blocked, the body has illness. Eastern medical practitioners have special placements to help unblock the energy that is causing hormonal imbalances. This is done by Naturopathic doctors or N.D.'s

Meditation is good for anything at any time your life, when things are going good or bad. Meditation helps you connect to your inner and higher source. It is like a form of prayer and helps to quiet the mind. Meditation can help you overcome the emotional hurdles with PCOS and may even help the body respond better to treatment by relieving stress. It is a deep form of relaxation and many people fall asleep during meditation sessions. In my companion book, I will have tips on how to meditate, breathing techniques and use of music and aromatherapy to increase the experience.

Herbal Therapies Herbal practitioners have herbal tonics that can help to balance the hormones in the body. It is extremely important to discuss these with your doctor before taking them and check for any drug interactions before using them with prescription medications. The upside to herbal therapies is side-effects can be little to none and they are often very effective. Just make sure you find a competent practitioner that is skilled in working with herbal therapies for PCOS so you can make sure you are on the right combination.

Traditional Chinese Medicine (TCM) Traditional Chinese medicine for PCOS focuses on the core body systems that could be causing the hormonal dysfunction. It starts by looking at the kidneys and the balances of yin/yang or female/male energies.

Treatment is usually diet that is low on the glycemic index with strict avoidance of sugar and Chinese herbal supplements that can help to balance hormones naturally. It also stresses the importance of yoga and meditation.

Ayurvedic Medicine This is the traditional medicine of India. It focuses on diet and herbal therapies to help balance the hormones. Most of the Ayurvedic treatments and herbs are already food based, so there is little chance of interactions or side-effects. It is still important to check herbs used in cooking food when you're on prescription medication. For example; cinnamon is used to control blood sugar, but may increase the effects of metformin and drop your blood sugar too low. Ayurvedic medicine also stresses the use of yoga and meditation.

Alternative Diets Some people try Vegetarian and Vegan diets in hopes that cutting animal products will improve hormonal balances. It is important to remember that we need to make sure we are not robbing our bodies of needed nutrients at this time. If you choose an alternative diet, make sure you consult a good book or nutritionist to help with your diet plan.

Most medical doctors are aware of Alternative medical treatments and more and more are becoming supportive of these approaches. When choosing a doctor, it will be helpful to ask how they feel about alternative treatments. This way you will know if you will be comfortable with your provider and that they will allow you to be a partner in planning your care.

The Ultimate Question: Will Treatment Work?

No matter what you choose and how good your specialist is, you will still constantly ask the question "Is it going to work?" The good news is that the anti-diabetic medications usually take care of the hyperinsulinemia and lower the androgens and most often, yes this treatment works very well. Fertility is a whole different story. Whether or not your ovaries choose to respond to the anti-diabetic medication is entirely up to them. At this point, they become their own little entity within your body and sometimes they have a mind of their own.

If you suffered from PCOS for long enough you may suffer from ovarian atrophy and premature ovarian failure. This is caused by excessive levels of testosterone and elevated glucose levels. This is what the surgeons found when they did my hysterectomy and removed my right ovary. It had completely atrophied and turned to stone. If I had only received a correct and proper diagnosis early enough this may not have happened. My left ovary must have been working, because after I started treatment with the anti-diabetic medication I became pregnant very quickly with my fourth child. Surprise! This is why getting a referral to a reproductive endocrinologist is of extreme importance as soon as you recognize the symptoms of PCOS.

The one thing that I can tell you is that once you begin eating healthy, exercising, and keep up with your treatment plan you will start to feel a lot better. Your energy levels are going to increase and your moods should stabilize. I know after I started treatment I lost about eighty pounds and I slowly started to resume normal activities that I hadn't done in a long time. I started accepting invitations to friend's houses, taking my kids out on more outings, and generally just living life like I should.

The one downside is some of the characteristics have not completely disappeared for me. Once in a while, my loving partner still plucks a stray chin hair or two. My body type is still "apple shaped" and I still have some cysts on my left ovary. My blood sugar and blood pressure are under very good control, but the condition still lingers somewhere in the background somewhere. I suppose that I have just adjusted to the "new me." It is less of a bother now.

COMPLIANCE IS THE KEY TO SUCCESS

Once you design your treatment plan, you have to stick to it. Eat the rabbit food, it's good for you. I never wanted to see another green leafy veggie again after I started my PCOS diet. It was grainy, leafy, and tasted bland. I wanted fast-food, potato chips and ice cream. Yes, I cheated on the diet once in a while. For the most part I forced myself to eat healthy foods and learned to cook with herbs, spices and condiments that would make the food taste better but not compromise my health.

Keep all of your doctor's appointments. Staying in touch with your doctor is very important. You also need to keep up with checking your blood sugar at least twice daily if you are on anti-diabetic medication. Your blood sugar may drop suddenly and you need to know what to do. Symptoms of low blood sugar include:

- ▶ Sweating
- ▶ Shakiness
- ▶ Confusion
- ▶ Agitation
- ▶ Lightheadedness
- ▶ Hunger
- ▶ Insomnia

▶ Headache

▶ Weakness

You also need to keep any and all lab appointments during treatment. Your doctor is going to periodically check your insulin levels, blood sugar levels, Hemoglobin A1C, and androgen levels. You may also have periodic ultrasounds to check your ovaries for cysts. I was checked about every six weeks when my cysts were active and painful. The doctor will watch to make sure they go down. It is not fun when they rupture, that's for sure!

If you are undergoing fertility treatments, it is going to be extremely important to take the medications exactly as prescribed by the doctor. The hormones you will be given are designed to work in cycles. Missing doses or taking extra will only throw the cycle off and you will have to start all over again the next month. Here are some of the fertility drugs that are used in PCOS:

▶ **Clomid (clomiphene citrate)**

▶ **Lupron (leuprolide)**

▶ **Follistim (FSH)**

▶ **Antagon (GnRH)**

▶ **Pregnyl (hCG)**

▶ **And others depending on your specialist's preference**

These drugs work by stimulating the hormones that cause ovulation to happen. Research your drugs, girls. You need to know all of the side-effects, especially the risk of multiples. There is an increased risk of "Ovarian Hyper stimulation" and you could end up with twins, triplets or more. Your actual risk of twins with Clomid is only 10 percent and higher multiples only 1 percent. With the high cost of fertility treatments, you need to do everything exactly as the doctor orders.

When keeping a basal temperature chart, you need to be compliant every single day of the month. I will be outlining this in my companion book with specific instructions for success. You cannot miss a day of taking your temperature; you cannot move, get up, drink coffee, or brush your teeth. Any movement or drinking could throw your temperature off and you could miss the one important day that you are looking for. This is a very dedicated technique and must be done precisely to work. I remember many mornings waking up and thinking to myself, "Cofffeeeeee" only to remember that I needed to grab my thermometer first. This is where the supportive partner comes in to remind you to take your temperature while they go down and make the coffee for you (Insert smiley here).

Speaking of your partner; be sure to include them in your doctor's appointments, treatment plan and your day to day feelings about PCOS. Make sure to make ample time for your partner to talk about their feelings too. You may find yourself getting so caught up in being the PCOS patient; remember your partner is suffering with you. Keeping them in the loop will help relieve stress on both of you.

PCOS Treatments do work well if you actively participate in them. Taking your medications every day, as prescribed and sticking to your treatment plan greatly increases your state of health and your chances of getting pregnant. The earlier you start treatment in this disorder; you reduce the risk of permanent infertility due to ovarian atrophy. You also reduce the risk of severe health complications due to high blood sugar, cholesterol and high blood pressure. The more you stick to treatment, the closer you are to becoming a PCOS Survivor!

Chapter Six

PCOS: The Road To Recovery Is Long, But The Worth The Effort

There was one point in my illness that I thought to myself, "I will never be the same again. I will never feel as good as I did before." You know what, I was right! But things did get better for me.

Your body is changing every day and has been since the day you were born. Along the road of life, you have probably noticed subtle and sometimes not so subtle changes in your body. There are moments when you mourn the energetic old you. Then one day you noticed that you have adapted to the "new you." You know you aren't what you used to be, yet you try to do as much as you can. You strive to give yourself a quality of life at whatever level you are at.

At least that is what I have done for myself. Yes, I do feel better now than I did in the throes of PCOS. I'm not the same as I was before, but I have adapted. I told myself long ago that I would not let this condition confine me to the house or my bed. Regardless of how I feel every day, I still get up and get out and live.

I found that lying in bed does not make PCOS better. Skipping functions, parties, and events does not do anything for how I feel. I found that the more I did, the better I felt. Whether it was just the exercise of moving around or the emotional uplift, I did feel better pushing through it. You need to understand that you will not die from PCOS, at least now anyways. As bad as you feel some days, you aren't dying. I kept thinking I was and that I needed to lie still and save my energy. It only made me feel worse. The exercise will actually naturally help bring your blood sugar levels down and improve insulin response. It is the high blood sugars that make you feel fatigued. Fatigue can also be a side-effect of metformin. All I know is rest didn't help at all.

So, you will improve with treatment and you will feel somewhat better. The rest you will learn to adapt to. Just remember the more you pay attention to your treatment plan, your diet and your exercise the better you will feel. It is all up to you. And your body will adapt.

THE BENEFITS OF STICKING TO YOUR DIET

Whether it is pregnancy or lowering blood sugar, you will reap many benefits of sticking to the PCOS diet plan. First and foremost, you need to be on a lower glycemic index to help combat insulin resistance. Second, your hormone levels need balancing and diet can help keep your body functioning as best it can.

I am a huge believer in the theory that the chemicals in processed foods can tweak our endocrine and our immune system. My motto to both my patients and my friends is, "if you can't read and understand the label on your food, why would you put it in your body?" Once I started eating less processed foods and started cooking from scratch, I felt so much better. How can I explain it? You feel less toxic and cleaner inside and out.

According to the *Natural Resources Defense Council,* "an endocrine disruptor is a synthetic chemical that when absorbed by the body either mimics or blocks hormones and disrupts the body's normal functions." The main sources of endocrine disruptors are pesticides and PCB's found in plastic. This furthers the evidence that drinking water from plastic water bottles may not be safe. It is also harmful to heat food in plastic containers in the microwave. And all of these things can affect your partner and his sperm count, so both of you should eat the PCOS diet together if planning for pregnancy.

Now you don't have to go out and buy everything organic, just shop the perimeter of the store. That is where all the fresh foods are hiding!

Is Pregnancy Possible With PCOS?

The statistics for pregnancy after PCOS treatment are actually pretty good if you follow a good plan. This means catching the condition early before ovaries atrophy, getting started on a good diet, and possibly medication to treat insulin resistance. The sooner the better! Pregnancy rates in women that take metformin for PCOS are moderately high and when Clomid is added, the pregnancy rates almost quadruple.

The only drawback is that PCOS has a higher miscarriage rate, about 45 percent of pregnancies in PCOS patients end in miscarriage. The other risks are higher rate of pre-eclampsia (pregnancy induced high blood pressure and proteinuria) and gestational diabetes. There is also a higher rate of pre-term delivery and higher birth weight babies due to hyperglycemia. Two of my pregnancies were uncomplicated and two of them were high-risk. I had severe pre-eclampsia with my first daughter and gestational diabetes with my second daughter. My first daughter had to be delivered early and spent her first week of life on a ventilator.

One possible solution to the higher miscarriage rates is monitoring progesterone levels during pregnancy. However, low progesterone levels may be a sign that the pregnancy is not going to be a healthy one and miscarriage may be a matter of natural selection. Some women have benefitted from progesterone replacement in the early months of pregnancy, but not all do. Heck, most people are willing to try anything and I say, "why not?" Just understand that it may or may not work.

If natural conception is not possible, there is always the option of donor eggs and surrogate mothers. The actual incidence of this happening these days is less common due to the increased education and prompt treatment of PCOS. You hear less about the "test tube" baby and more mothers are able to conceive even if they need extensive fertility treatment.

The good thing about pregnancy with PCOS is after the birth of your baby you will experience a sort of PCOS "honeymoon phase." The hormones of pregnancy will help regulate your body and cycles for some time. You may even experience the lucky surprise of a second pregnancy during this time that happens without even trying. I think that is what happened between my second and third kids. I really had to try for my second child; PCOS diet, basal charting, etcetera. Then when she was a year old, I got pregnant with my third without even trying. My fourth was the result of PCOS treatment. Four kids with PCOS is a very good and positive number. Even one for some people is a blessing. I am just living proof that paying attention to details and treatment pays off!

WHERE DOES THE PCOS ROAD LEAD?

PCOS can lead you down many paths, it is your choice which one to take. If your desire is a healthy pregnancy and healthy baby, that will become your path. If you need to treat hyperglycemia, high blood pressure or high cholesterol, then that needs to be your focus. Your doctor will help you decide if it is the right time for pregnancy, or if you should stabilize your hormonal levels first. This is important to guarantee your pregnancy will be healthy. Being pregnant in the throes of PCOS without treatment could mean complications. I am convinced this is why I suffered pre-eclampsia so badly with my oldest daughter. I only used the diet with no other treatment. Sometimes nature shows us that we are not in charge of things. If you need to be treated for a while first, be patient it will pay off in the long run.

After all is said and done and you have started treatment and are maintaining your diet and you feel better, then you will truly be able to call yourself a PCOS survivor. Once this happens, you will find the tools to help yourself and possibly even the strength to help others down the road. It is important to remember; once you are a survivor that means that you have acquired the tools and the patience to deal with your condition. There is no cure for PCOS. Not even my hysterectomy was a cure. My body somewhere somehow still produces little extra androgens. It is less than it was before, but I am much better able to manage it overall.

I have mostly recovered from PCOS. I had four pregnancies. I don't really have blood sugar problems anymore. My blood pressure can run a little high sometimes and I get the occasional chin hair. My PCOS had actually been in remission for quite a few years. Lately, I have had a few challenges, but not too bad. Regardless, I call myself a PCOS survivor and my hope is that you can call yourself that someday too.

Conclusion

Closing Thoughts From Kim

Well, there it is in a little more than a nutshell. I have taken you through my personal experience with Polycystic Ovarian Syndrome. From suspecting I had PCOS, to lab testing, diagnosing and treatments, I enjoyed sharing my journey with you.

Let's look back at what we know now. You may be strongly suspicious that you have PCOS or you may have already been diagnosed. The important fact is to take a good long look at how you want to live with PCOS and decide on your plan of action from here. The best thing I can suggest is find a good reproductive endocrinologist for advice and help. Once you have seen a knowledgeable doctor, then tailor your plan with what works for you. Only you know in your heart what will be right and trying is your first step.

Understand that the lab tests, temperature charting, and treatments may be a very long road and it is important not to give up. It is okay to take a break from fertility attempts for a while, but keep going with treatment for any health conditions such as high blood sugar, high cholesterol, and high blood pressure. Medical conditions related to PCOS need to be monitored by a physician.

Lastly, watch for my upcoming companion books that will help guide you through treatment and diet in both medical and natural/holistic fields of medicine. Then you can tailor your approach to what suits you best, of course after checking with your physician. Learn how to chart temperatures, eat healthy, incorporate exercise and feel better about yourself with simple and easy to learn techniques.

Final Note: as I write these very last paragraphs, I am currently lying in a hospital bed. I just got the news that I have two 3 cm cysts on my remaining left ovary. I have a referral to a gynecologist and I may need to have the ovary removed. Somehow, I am not scared anymore. Somehow, I don't feel alone anymore. I see the light at the end of the tunnel. Hopefully, once the ovary is gone my androgen production will finally stabilize. During this time I have spent with you, helping you start your journey, I myself just got one step closer to the end of mine. And, somehow, in writing this book for you, you have helped me too! I want to thank each and every one of you for taking the time to read my book.

Please try to stay positive. Keep journaling your symptoms, your thoughts and keep track of what you eat daily. It is a long road, but just understand that just by reading a book on PCOS you are on the path to feeling better. This shows that you are brave and willing to fight and not let it get you down.

I invite you to join me on my Face Book page titled, **"Peach Fuzz and Baggage: PCOS From A Survivors Point Of View"**, and please feel free to send e-mails and correspondence.

Appendix

Education on PCOS
For Teens:
http://www.girlshealth.gov/parents/parentsbody/pcos_educators.cfm
http://www.youngwomenshealth.org
http://kidshealth.org/teen/sexual_health/girls/pcos.html
For Women:
http://www.pcosfoundation.org/about
http://www.soulcysters.com/
http://www.pcoschallenge.org/pcos-support/

Support Groups
http://www.pcosupport.org/
http://pcos.supportgroups.com/
http://www.pcoschallenge.org/pcos-support/

Clinical Trials
http://www.centerwatch.com/clinical-trials/listings/condition/313/
polycystic-ovarian-syndrome

Face Book Page
https://www.facebook.com/pages/You-and-Me-and-
PCOS/118914748286284
Fertility Resources
http://attainfertility.com/
http://www.resolve.org/

http://www.resolve.org/support-and-services/
http://www.fertilehope.org/tool-bar/referral-guide-about.cfm

Resources
I would like to thank all of the following publications, websites, fellow survivors, and PCOS researchers for all of their hard work in helping us to fight this disorder. Our success as survivors is because of all your hard work:

http://pullingdownthemoon.com/fertility/pcos-and-cortisol-why-a-relaxation-regimen-is-not-optional/
http://www.ncbi.nlm.nih.gov/pubmed/20528321
http://www.ncbi.nlm.nih.gov/pubmed/17558682 PCOS/PGA relationship
http://www.ncbi.nlm.nih.gov/pmc/articles/PMC2366795/ PCOS and Vitamins
http://www.medscape.com/viewarticle/522390 Lifestyle modifications
http://women.webmd.com/tc/polycystic-ovary-syndrome-pcos-medications
http://humupd.oxfordjournals.org/content/13/3/249.short Surgery
http://www.mayoclinic.com/health/polycystic-ovary-syndrome/DS00423/DSECTION=complications
http://womenshealth.about.com/cs/pcos/a/whatispcos.htm
http://www.nlm.nih.gov/medlineplus/ency/article/000369.htm
http://www.ivf.com/pcostreat.html
http://www.ncbi.nlm.nih.gov/pubmedhealth/PMH0001502/
http://www.cedars-sinai.edu/Patients/Programs-and-Services/Androgen-Related-Research-and-Discovery-Center/Symptoms-and-Diagnosis/Irregular-Menstrual-Periods.aspx
http://www.ncbi.nlm.nih.gov/pubmedhealth/PMH0004546/
http://europepmc.org/abstract/MED/16682845/reload=0;jsessionid=Mg76jYNoi3yGti1ujzZ0.16
http://clinical.diabetesjournals.org/content/21/4/154.full
http://www.mayoclinic.com/health/medical/IM03929

http://womenshealth.gov/publications/our-publications/fact-sheet/
polycystic-ovary-syndrome.cfm
http://informahealthcare.com/doi/abs/10.1080/09513590312331290268
http://www.ncbi.nlm.nih.gov/pubmed/17044949
http://nurse-practitioners-and-physician-assistants.advanceweb.com/
SharedResources/Downloads/2010/012510/NP020110_p18table1.pdf
http://onlinelibrary.wiley.com/doi/10.1002/ar.1092110410/abstract
http://www.nrdc.org/health/effects/qendoc.asp
http://pcosfoundation.org/support-groups?gclid=COmlu8rC7bQCFdKd
4AodJiwAnw
http://www.brainyquote.com/quotes/keywords/alone.html
http://www.ncbi.nlm.nih.gov/pubmed/20802269
http://www.nhlbi.nih.gov/guidelines/obesity/e_txtbk/txgd/4142.htm
http://www.ncbi.nlm.nih.gov/pubmed/8291455
http://www.ncbi.nlm.nih.gov/pubmed/14671189
http://jcem.endojournals.org/content/92/3/787.long
http://www.hormone.org/endo101/
http://www.ncbi.nlm.nih.gov/pubmed/21835833
http://www.medscape.com/viewarticle/773342_2
http://psychcentral.com/archives/support_groups.htm

The Lancet (2007, September 3). Polycystic Ovary Syndrome: 1 In 15
Women Affected Worldwide And Burden Likely To Increase.

Images:

Figure 1: Endocrine System

www.epa.gov

Figure 2: Apple-Pear Body Type

www.womenshealth.gov

Figure 3: Normal Menstrual Cycle

www.yalemedicalgroup.org

Figure 4: Sample Basal Temperature Chart

www.library.med.utah.edu

Figure 5: The Cycle of Insulin Resistance

www.edrv.endojournals.org

About the Author

Kimberly Davis is a forty-four year old mother of two sons; ages twenty-seven and thirteen, and two daughters ages fifteen and six. She is also grandmother to two grandsons. Kimberly lived with PCOS for most of her adult life and still suffers the effects today. Yet, she calls herself a PCOS survivor and chooses to live a full and happy life. Kimberly just recently relocated from California to New England to fulfill her lifelong dream of becoming a writer. She is a retired Licensed Vocational Nurse and currently works as an Innkeeper at a quaint little New England Bed and Breakfast. She lives with her 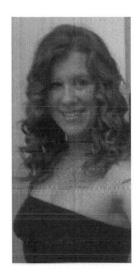 fiancé and childhood friend of thirty years and her two daughters.

Kimberly chooses to write from a medical and survivor's perspective in order to relate and form connections and bonds with other sufferers of PCOS. She has also started a related support group on the popular social networking site Facebook. It is her deepest concern that those who suffer from misunderstood conditions get little support and understanding.

Watch for more books she is working on in the health related field and also her first novel; a memoir of her childhood and reunion with her childhood sweetheart to be published soon.

"Has PCOS been a source of torment in your life and you're ready to fight?" Kimberly offers uplifting quotes and coping skills to help build your strength.

"Have you tried to deal with PCOS on your own and nothing worked?" You have come to the right place. Sharing her techniques for surviving this condition, she reaches out to women who may feel lost and alone in their battle.

"You had a sneaking suspicion that PCOS was causing your health issues." This book summarizes signs of this condition to share with your doctor. There are also helpful links included for more information and resources to get help along the way.

"Stand with me as I guide you down the road to becoming a survivor!" This book helps you connect and create a foundation of knowledge to begin living as a PCOS Survivor, from a very down to earth perspective.

Made in the USA
Lexington, KY
19 May 2014